Taking Control of Your Healthcare

Providing You and Your Loved Ones with the Information You Need to Participate in Your Care

Jeffrey I. Kreisberg, Ph.D.,
Suzanne H. Kreisberg, M.D.,
Lawrence M. Kreisberg, M.S.,
Joan M. Kreisberg, M.S.

iUniverse, Inc.
New York   Bloomington

Taking Control of Your Healthcare
Providing You and Your Loved Ones with the Information
You Need to Participate in Your Care

Copyright © 2009 Jeffrey Kreisberg

The information, ideas, and suggestions in this book are not intended
as a substitute for professional medical advice. Before following any
suggestions contained in this book, you should consult your personal
physician. Neither the author nor the publisher shall be liable or responsible
for any loss or damage allegedly arising as a consequence of your use
or application of any information or suggestions in this book.

iUniverse books may be ordered through booksellers or by contacting:

iUniverse
1663 Liberty Drive
Bloomington, IN 47403
www.iuniverse.com
1-800-Authors (1-800-288-4677)

Because of the dynamic nature of the Internet, any Web addresses or
links contained in this book may have changed since publication and
may no longer be valid. The views expressed in this work are solely those
of the author and do not necessarily reflect the views of the publisher,
and the publisher hereby disclaims any responsibility for them.

ISBN: 978-1-4401-7122-2 (pbk)
ISBN: 978-1-4401-7124-6 (cloth)
ISBN: 978-1-4401-7123-9 (ebk)

Printed in the United States of America

iUniverse rev. date: 10/02/09

Contents

Introduction

The greatest mistake in the treatment of diseases is that there are physicians for the body and physicians for the soul, although the two cannot be separated.

—Plato

Each day across America, people are misdiagnosed or receive incorrect information about their healthcare.

When was the last time you asked your doctor specific questions about the treatment he recommended? Perhaps you have handled your medical life and healthcare decisions with blind trust, or perhaps you're someone who likes to do their research on the Internet and ask a lot of questions. If you're in the latter category, it could be something that saves your life.

For example, Jane was a forty-year-old woman who had been told she had to have major and risky surgery after a carotid artery scan revealed an 80 percent blockage. "You have to do this surgery," the doctor said. "It's not optional. At your age, you are taking too much risk not to do it."

Jane and her husband were devastated at the thought of it. The surgery was very invasive, and they had two young daughters. They left the doctor's office in tears, feeling helpless. But then they decided to take charge of their healthcare and get a second opinion. Weeks later, after many sleepless nights, another scan revealed completely normal results. The artery was not blocked at all! This second opinion saved Jane from what could have been a life-threatening surgery and hospital stay. It could have meant the difference between life and death.

Research has shown that when medical decision making shifts from "delegated" to "shared," you are more likely to follow your doctor's instructions and pay closer attention to your care.[1,2] "Delegated" decision making is when

---

1 nahq.org/journal/ce/article.html?article_id=168.
2 pubmedcentral.nih.gov/articlerender.fcgi?tool=pubmed&pubmedid=16405711.

the doctor proclaims what your care will be and you have no recourse but to follow his or her instructions. However, in order to effectively participate in your healthcare, you have to get smart and have the necessary information to make an informed decision. My co-authors and I have the necessary experience in medical research, healthcare, and mental health to provide you with the information you need to participate in your healthcare.

I am a scientist and medical educator and together with my pathologist wife, Suzanne, and my brother and sister-in-law, Larry and Joan Kreisberg, who are both mental health professionals, we provide you with over a hundred years of experience in healthcare to help you get the information you need to navigate our complicated healthcare system. We provide you with guidelines to follow and arm you with important questions to ask your doctor so he can make the right diagnosis and you can make an informed decision, approaching your care as a team.

Approximately 15 percent of all patients are misdiagnosed, which results in serious harm to about half of them.[3] As discussed by Dr. Jerome Groopman, author of *How Doctors Think*, most doctor errors are due to mistakes in their thinking.[4] Doctors can make mistakes because of snap judgments based on the first symptom, physical finding, or lab value, or by stereotyping. For example, a woman comes in complaining of anxiety. The doctor may attribute this symptom to hysteria (the so-called hysterical female), when in fact the symptoms may be a sign of a heart attack. Therefore, it's most important to provide your doctor with all the information she needs to make an accurate diagnosis and to ask the right questions so she can focus her attention on you.

We've identified key areas for you to understand so you can take control of your healthcare. The book is organized into two parts. The first part addresses general healthcare issues; the second part addresses leading illnesses. In chapter 1, we focus on the doctor's appointment, indicating which questions you can ask and how to conduct yourself during the office visit. In subsequent chapters, we tell you how to take control of your hospital stay (chapter 2), your medication (chapter 3), and your health insurance (chapter 4). We've included a chapter for taking control of your health specifically for seniors (chapter 5) and one that shows how to take control and manage chronic disease (chapter 6). Finally, we review how your emotions can affect your health (chapter 14). Specific considerations for pediatric patients are also examined. In the

---

3 Newman-Tucker DE, Pronovost PJ. "Diagnostic Errors The Next Frontier for Patient Safety" JAMA 301: 1060, 2009.

4 Jerome Groopman, M.D. *How Doctors think*, Houghton Mifflin Harcourt: Boston, 2007.

appendix, we've included important Web sites and phone numbers you can use to get the information you need to take control of your healthcare.

One piece of advice we give throughout this book is to get a second opinion, especially after a diagnosis of cancer. Allow us to share a story from our practice. Melinda called us after she found out that she had breast cancer. She had a biopsy of a lump in her breast that was found after a mammogram. Needless to say she was shaken up. We encouraged her to relax. If indeed she did have breast cancer, there were now terrific treatments for a cure, we said. But first, she had to get a second opinion. Breast cancer is not easy to diagnose if the pathologist doesn't examine many such cases in his practice; therefore, we recommended a pathologist who was the world authority on breast cancer. He disagreed with the original diagnosis and said she did not have breast cancer. This information was invaluable to Melinda. Not only did she avoid the costs of treatment and lost wages, but she spared herself the risks associated with a possible mastectomy and the radiation and chemotherapy that go along breast cancer treatment.

In another instance, Gary was diagnosed with early-stage prostate cancer, and his urologist recommended immediate radical prostatectomy (removal of prostate and lymph nodes). He called us and we recommended getting a second opinion, referring him to a pathologist with expertise in prostate cancer. This time the second opinion agreed with the original diagnosis. We then told him there were many treatment options available to him, and we recommended he speak with a urologist who was an internationally recognized authority on prostate cancer treatment. Gary traveled 1200 miles for the consultation we arranged and was advised to hold off on surgery and to keep vigilance over his cancer by repeating the biopsy every six months. That was five years ago and the cancer has not grown. These patients from all over the country come to our patient advocacy service to get the information they need to get the right care.[5]

Much of what doctors do is based more on hunches rather than on what is called evidence-based medicine. Evidence-based medicine has emerged as a way to improve and evaluate patient care. It is largely based applying on the best scientific evidence available in combination with the patient's preferences, concerns, and expectations. This allows doctors and patients to form a partnership that optimizes clinical outcomes and quality of life. Evidence-based medicine has resulted in the development of best-practice guidelines to evaluate and treat patients with similar medical conditions. Unfortunately, today, doctors still over-treat patients and ignore best-practice guidelines.

A good example of the practice of medicine getting away from evidence-

---

5   KreisbergandAssociates.com.

based medicine can be seen in the number of inappropriate angioplasties done each year in this country. In an angioplasty, a balloon is used to open a clogged blood vessel in the heart. There are about two million angioplasties performed in the United States each year; 800,000 have been proven necessary, based on the prevailing scientific evidence. That is, the practice guidelines developed from evidence-based medicine show that angioplasties should only be performed in patients who are having a heart attack. The remaining 1,200,000 angioplasties were elective surgeries; 160,000 were found to be inappropriate, and 500,000 were of questionable value.[6] If you knew the risks involved with the procedure, would you have had the angioplasty? The purpose of this book is to give you the information you need to be an *effective partner* with your doctor in your healthcare so you get the right care.

Some Common Myths about Our Healthcare Systems

There are many myths about our healthcare system, myths that lead people into accepting diagnoses and treatments that aren't correct or necessary. We have all heard many of these myths, things we take for granted because they come from what we believe to be reputable sources. In order to get smart about your healthcare, it is important to understand the differences between myth and fact.

Myth 1: The United States has the best healthcare system in the world.
Fact: The United States ranks near the bottom among industrialized countries in infant mortality and adult life expectancy, two measurements of the quality of our healthcare system. What we do have, however, is the most expensive healthcare system. Incredibly, despite the costs of our healthcare, we get on average only 50 percent of the healthcare we need. [7,8]

Due to our lack of attention to preventive care, we have a growing problem of chronic disease. One in two Americans (125 million) suffers from one or more chronic diseases, such as heart disease, diabetes, cancer, pulmonary disease, Alzheimer's disease, hypertension, and stroke. Many of these diseases are preventable. Chronic disease accounts for seven of every ten deaths (1.7 million) each year! People with chronic diseases represent all segments of society. More than 75 percent of people with chronic conditions are under

---

6   Shannon Brownlee, *Overtreated*, Bloomsbury: New York, 2007.

7   S. A. Schroeder, "We Can Do Better: Improving the Health of the American People," *NEJM* 357:1221, 2007.

8   Robert Wood Johnson Foundation, rwjf.org/files/publications/other/asch_nejm_20060316.pdf.

the age of sixty-five, while 80 percent of senior Americans live with at least one chronic disease, and 50 percent have two![9]

In the Medicare population, the average beneficiary sees more than seven different physicians and fills upwards of fifteen medications.[10,11] Since the population of Americans sixty-five and older is expected to double in the next twenty-five years, we must not only make sure people with chronic diseases receive the right care, but we must also do something to prevent chronic disease from occurring.

Myth 2: All medications are safe because they have been approved by the Food and Drug Administration (FDA).
Fact: In reality, 400,000 people are hurt or killed each year because either they receive the wrong drug or dose of drug or there is a serious interaction between drugs and between drugs and dietary supplements.[12]

Myth 3: Over-the-counter medications are safe.
Fact: This is true as long as you follow the directions in the "Drug Facts" box on the package label. Be aware that many cold products contain acetaminophen (Tylenol) so be sure not to take Tylenol as a pain reliever when on these medications. This will cause double-dosing of pain reliever.

There is also a common misconception that generic drugs are not as safe or effective as their brand-name counterparts. Generic drugs are subjected to the same FDA requirements as brand names and are safe, effective, and less expensive than brand-name drugs. Use them with confidence.

Myth 4: Hospitals are the safest place to be when you're sick.
Fact: This is perhaps the greatest myth of all. Please don't misunderstand. Hospitals play a critical role in healthcare. However, there are more than one million preventable adverse events in hospitals each year in the United States, of which 98,000 are fatal.[13] Some leading culprits are wrong site surgery, leaving operating materials (such as sponges) in patients, medication error, and operative or post-operative complications.

So, how did we get in such a mess? It is largely the result of the diseases that usually cause acute illness (for example, diabetes, hypertension, and heart disease) becoming chronic conditions because of the lack of monitoring and

---

9   fightchronicdisease.com/issues/about.cfm.
10 nationalprioritiespartnership.org/PriorityDetails.aspx?id=606.
11 ashp.org/import/news/HealthSystemPharmacyNews/newsarticle.aspx?id=1956.
12 annals.org/cgi/reprint/140/1/33.pdf.
13 "To Err is Human" Institute of Medicine, Quality of Healthcare in America, 1999.

treatment. This happens, in part, because the healthcare industry in the United States today is overspecialized, with fewer primary care doctors to provide yearly check-ups and because the care they offer is not coordinated across providers and service settings. The primary care doctor plays a prominent role in the diagnosis, treatment, and management of disease. Since there does not appear to be much hope of more practicing primary care physicians in the near future, we have to make lifestyle changes to prevent and manage disease so we and our loved ones receive the right care.

Here is the good news. While this book will uncover many myths and potentially disturbing facts about the current state of healthcare, its purpose is to educate you so that you are equipped to make the right decisions about your own welfare and help your loved ones make better decisions for ourselves.

PART 1
Taking Control of Your Health

Chapter One

Take Control of Your Doctor's Appointment

Objectives:
- Provide you with tips on finding the right doctor
- Provide you with tips on preparing for your doctor's appointment
- Provide you with questions to ask while at the doctor's office so you get the right care

Actual Case: Our father was diagnosed with prostate cancer when he was fifty-two years old, and the urologist recommended immediate surgery. I told him there was no hurry for surgery, because prostate cancer was slow growing. Instead, I had him send his biopsy to me (Dr. Jeffrey Kreisberg) so I could have my colleagues in the Department of Pathology give a second opinion. Twelve pathologists examined the biopsy and none could find any cancer. The director of surgical pathology at the medical school recommended that Dad have his biopsy repeated in six months. He did and it was negative. So were the next six biopsies. Dad died of heart failure when was eighty-three years old. The take-home message is that in order to receive the right care, you must find the right doctor, find the right hospital, and **GET A SECOND OPINION!**

More Myths about the Healthcare System

Myth: Americans receive all the care they need for their disease.

Fact: Americans receive only about half the recommended healthcare they need.[14] The USA has the highest rate of preventable deaths among nineteen industrialized countries.[15]

Myth: I am young and healthy. I don't need to see a doctor.

Fact: It is important for maintaining good health to visit your doctor annually. Preventive screening for diseases such as diabetes, heart disease, and sexually transmitted diseases is important for maintaining health; likewise, so are immunizations to prevent disease. Eighty percent of preventive care occurs during other kinds of office visits, such as appointments for a minor ailment.

Finding the Right Doctor

In order to receive the right care, the patient and the physician must be cooperatively involved in the management of healthcare with the goal being high-quality, cost-effective medical care. This is best accomplished with a primary care physician who is trained in General Internal Medicine, Family Medicine (adults), or Pediatrics (children up until eighteen years of age). Primary care physicians coordinate your care with other consulting specialties so you receive the best care. Coordinated care prevents duplication of care and ensures all specialists are on the same page.

> **To find a primary-care doctor, go to the American Board of Medical Specialties (abms.org). To do a check-up on your doctor, go to healthgrades.com, or ucomparehealth. com.**

If you have problems locating a doctor you like, consider trying the following:

- Call your local hospitals. They often have free physician-referral services and can tell you which doctors have hospital privileges or are taking new patients.
- Work your way through your insurer's list of physicians. Unfortunately, these lists are often out of date, and it can take hours of calling to find doctors who are accepting patients. If you continue to have

---

14 The Robert Wood Johnson Foundation, at rwjf.org/files/publications/other/asch_nejm_20060316.pdf.

15 pnhp.org/news/2008/january/us_has_most_preven.php.

problems, call the benefits office at your place of employment or the customer service department of your insurance provider.

- For routine care (such as strep-throat tests, flu shots, and pneumococcal vaccines), consider visiting an ambulatory urgent care center or one of the retail clinics in pharmacies, discount department, and grocery stores. They're often open nights and weekends, and are particularly appealing to younger patients, people who don't have chronic illnesses, and the uninsured.

You will know if you made the right choice in a doctor if you feel comfortable talking to him about your medical condition.

Good doctors should listen attentively to your concerns, allowing you to speak without interruption.

Importantly, they should spend time with you, explaining the reasons behind their treatment or medication decisions. You should feel like an equal and never as if are you being talked down to. If the office staff is rude or unhelpful, report this to the doctor. *A good relationship with your doctor and her staff allows you to participate in your healthcare and is the key to a successful outcome!*

Be Prepared for Your Examination

Before your visit, *call for instructions.* Ask when you make your appointment whether the doctor will be performing any laboratory tests at your appointment. Some laboratory tests require you to fast (skip breakfast) for the test to be accurate. If you must fast, you may want to consider a morning appointment.

Gather and take with you all lab reports, X-rays, and contact information for any specialists you're seeing. In addition, know your family medical history. Many medical conditions, such as hypertension, heart disease, and diabetes, run in families. It is important for you to know the medical history of your parents as well as your grandparents. You should also know the cause of death of any deceased family members.

Lastly, fill out and carry with you at all times the *Pill Card* shown in the appendix. This provides you space to list all your prescription and non-prescription medications and dietary supplements. This list is also important to have on you in medical emergency situations.

At the Doctor's Office

As you know, doctors are overworked and under a lot of stress, which can lead to mistakes. Approximately 15 percent of all patients are misdiagnosed, which results in serious harm to about half of them.[16] Most errors made by doctors are due to three common mistakes in their thinking:

1. Making snap judgments based on the first symptom, physical finding, or lab value.
2. Rendering a diagnosis based on symptoms and physical findings typical of other recently seen cases but that don't apply to yours.
3. Stereotyping individuals and attributing symptoms to this stereotype. For example, a woman complaining of shortness of breath and neck, upper back, shoulder, or jaw pain may be diagnosed as having anxiety, but she could really be having a heart attack!

The next thing you need to be prepared for is paperwork. There are pages of medical history to fill out, as well as a privacy statement to sign. The authors recommend showing up thirty minutes before your appointment time. If you have questions about filling out the paperwork, ask one of the office staff.

When you fill out your medical history, answer all the questions truthfully. List the amount of alcohol you drink, the cigarettes you smoke, and any recreational drugs you use. Your medical record is private and cannot, by law, be released to anyone without your permission. Hiding the truth can be dangerous, because there are prescription medications that interact with other drugs, alcohol, or recreational drugs in a life-threatening manner.

Filling out the paperwork truthfully is the best way to ensure you get the right care. You are the only one who will suffer the consequences of withholding crucial medical information. For example, by withholding information about your alcohol intake, you are denying the doctor important information he needs to safely prescribe medications that may interact with alcohol. Your medical history is protected under the HIPAA Privacy Rule, so be honest about it. The Privacy Rule absolutely prohibits healthcare providers and plans from disclosing personal health information to employers without a patient's explicit, written authorization.

---

16 D. E. Newman-Tucker and P. J. Pronovost, "Diagnostic Errors: The Next Frontier for Patient Safety," *JAMA* 301: 1060, 2009.

Ask the Right Questions

In order to receive the right care it is important to participate in your treatment. To do so, you must be informed. Below, we provide you with some questions to ask your provider that will give you the information you need to participate in your care, which is key to receiving the right care.

There are questions you can ask the doctor so his attention is focused on you, the patient. *To help prevent a mistake in diagnosis, always ask the following*:

1. What is my diagnosis (the medical name for the illness I have), and what does it mean?
2. What else could the diagnosis be?
3. Could more than one thing be going on to explain my symptoms?
4. Is there anything is my history, physical exam, or test results that does not fit into your diagnosis?
5. How serious is my diagnosis?
6. What treatments are recommended?
7. Are there other treatment options? What are they? Often times there are less expensive, safer alternative treatments or drugs that could be prescribed.
8. What benefits can I expect from the recommended treatments and other options?
9. What are the risks or complications of the recommended treatment and the other treatment options?
10. Will the treatment cause any discomfort?
11. What methods will be used to prevent or relieve these discomforts?
12. What are the side effects of the treatment—immediate, short-term, and long-term?
13. How will having treatment affect my normal functions and everyday activities?
14. How would not having treatment affect my normal functions and everyday activities?
15. How long will treatment last?
16. How long will it be before I can go back to my normal activities?
17. How much does the treatment cost? The 2008 Kaiser Health Tracking Poll revealed that nearly half the public (47 percent) reported someone in their family skipping pills, postponing, or cutting back on medical care due to the cost of care.[17] Often, expensive is not

---

17 Kaiser Family Foundation, at kff.org/kaiserpolls/h08_posr102108pkg.cfm.

better.[18] In fact, expensive procedures are often more risky, and there may be medical alternatives that are safer and cheaper. Discuss other options with your doctor.

You have the right to refuse treatment and the doctor is morally obligated to provide you with the information you need to make that decision.

If your doctor recommends testing:
18. Are there any foods or drinks I should avoid before or after the test?
19. When will I be notified about the results of the test? Don't assume that no news is good news. Many mistakes are made because test results get lost. Most of these are caused by communication breakdowns.

If you leave with a prescription, make sure your doctor wrote it for the right drug and gave you instructions on when and how to take it as well as its side effects. Ask if you should be concerned about drug interactions with any of the medications and dietary *supplements you are taking. Confirm this with the pharmacist when you pick up your medication.*

The Importance of a Second Opinion

You should always get a second opinion if,

* You are diagnosed with cancer
* You are uncomfortable or feel uninformed about your course of treatment
* You are agreeing to elective surgery

In 30 percent of cases where patients voluntarily seek a second opinion for elective surgery, and in 18 percent of cases where an insurance company requires a second opinion, the second opinion does not confirm the original diagnosis.[19]

You can ask your doctor to recommend someone for a second opinion. You can go to the following Web sites for help locating a doctor for a second

18 K. Balcker and A. Chandra, "Medicare Spending, the Physician Workforce, and Beneficiaries Quality of Care," Health Affairs Web exclusive W4 184-197, 2008.
19 nytimes.com/2008/02/12/health/views/12essa.html?_r=1&bl&ex=1203051600 &en=bf8812ecc5524a95&ei=5087 percent0A.

opinion: abms.org, healthgrades.com, or ucomparehealth.com. A medical school is a good place to find a doctor for a second opinion. Call the appropriate department at the school for your treatment. Many insurance companies cover the costs of second opinions; consult your insurance company's brochure.

Make sure you understand everything that you need to know before signing an informed consent (see below).

Four Signs of an Unsafe Practice[20]

After your visit, ask yourself questions to evaluate your doctor. If your doctor is operating an unsafe practice, find another doctor. Here are four signs to look for:

1. The doctor doesn't listen to you.
2. The doctor's technology is in the dark ages. For example, you are less safe if your doctor uses paper recordkeeping than electronic records. You shouldn't have to fill out the same paperwork every time you visit the doctor; rather, they should be asking you whether anything has changed in your health status and using this information to update your electronic medical record.
3. Your doctor fails to contact you with test results even once.
4. Other patients have complained.

Informed Consent

When you seek medical care, you usually talk with the doctor to get her recommendations about the next step in your treatment. Most people follow these recommendations, but you are not required to do so. If you are an adult who is able to make your own decisions, you are the only person who can choose which course of action to take.

In order to get the right care, patients and their families are becoming partners in their healthcare.

All medical care requires the informed consent of the patient (or an appointed guardian) before the care plan is carried out. In some cases, you approve the doctor's plan by simply getting a prescription filled, allowing

---

20 Lorie Parch, "Danger at Your Doctor's Office," *Health*, September 2008.

blood to be drawn for lab tests, or seeing a specialist. This is called simple consent, and is okay for treatments that carry little risk for you.

In cases where there are larger possible risks, you may be asked to agree in writing to the doctor's plan for your care. *Informed consent* recognizes your need to know about a procedure, surgery, or treatment before you decide to have it. The answers to the questions suggested above should provide you with the information you need to provide informed consent.

Informed consent is a process in which,

- You are told about the possible risks and benefits of the treatment.
- You are informed of the risks and benefits of other options, including not getting treatment.
- You have the chance to ask questions and receive satisfactory answers.
- You have had time (if needed) to discuss the plan with family or advisors.
- You are able to use the information to help make an informed decision that you think is in your own best interest.
- You communicate that decision to your doctor or treatment team.

As mentioned earlier, a competent adult cannot be forced to take any type of medical treatment. In general, anything other than a life-threatening emergency, in which the patient is unconscious, requires consent before treatment. Even in that situation, consent may sometimes be required if the patient is known to have an advanced directive (for example, a do-not-resuscitate order, or DNR).

Remember, it is your right to not give consent or to seek another opinion.

Who Besides the Patient Can Give Consent?

For children or others who are unable to make their own decisions, the parent or legal guardian is legally responsible for getting the information, making the decision, and signing the consent form. Along the same lines, people who are unable to manage their daily affairs due to mild dementia (impaired thinking) or emotional problems may still be able to understand the medical situation and make their wishes known.

> **The main purpose of the informed consent process is to protect you, the patient.**

In the event that you are unable to take in information and make your wishes known, another person may be called upon to take part in the process of informed consent. *One way to have a voice in choosing this person is to designate a durable power of attorney for healthcare* (also called a medical power of attorney; more about Advanced Directives such as durable power of attorney is discussed in chapter 5, "Take Control of Your Health—for Seniors.") If you are unable to speak for yourself because of illness or disability, the person you chose becomes legally responsible for making medical decisions on your behalf. This person is sometimes called your proxy, agent, or surrogate.

In the absence of a medical power of attorney the court may appoint a guardian, surrogate, or proxy to make medical decisions for you. If you become unable to make decisions for yourself, someone else—such as the doctor, the facility, a friend, or a family member—may petition the court to appoint someone to do it for you. The process varies from state to state.

Many states have passed *family agency acts* that choose which family members (in a listed order of priority) may act on behalf of a person who cannot speak for himself. This is likely only if you do not have an advanced directive or court-appointed proxy. Depending on your family situation and your state of health, that person may be your legal guardian, spouse, parent, child, sibling, or other relative.

Consent forms stipulate that you have the right to stop a long course of treatment or withdraw from a study even if you have already signed a consent form. Even if the form does not mention it, you still have this right. In this case, you need to contact the doctor in charge of your treatment (or of the clinical trial) to make your wishes known. You may be asked to sign a form refusing further treatment so that the doctor or facility will have a legal record.

What Is the Process of Informed Consent for Enrolling in a Clinical Trial?

Enrolling in a clinical trial usually involves more information than the consent form for any standard treatment. The informed consent process should tell you what the clinical trial is set up to find out, what is expected of you, what the expected benefits are, what is known and not known about the new drug or procedure, and other possible treatment options.

Before you make your decision, the research team will talk with you about the clinical trial's purpose, procedures, risks, and possible benefits, as well as your rights as a participant. If you decide to participate, the team will continue to update you on any new information that may affect you and your situation. Before, during, and even after the trial, you will have the chance to ask questions and voice your concerns. Informed consent for clinical trials goes on for as long as the research lasts, and even afterward.

> **You must realize that a clinical trial is research; it is unproven and nonstandard treatment. Its purpose is to benefit future patients; any benefits to you are uncertain.**

Take *an* advocate with you if you become anxious at doctor's appointments and cannot effectively participate in your care. Your advocate should review the important questions you want answered by the doctor and review the answers with you after the appointment. A professional advocate will educate you about your diagnosis and the treatment options recommended by your doctor.

1. Make sure you ask the doctor, or one of his staff, for a form giving consent for your advocate to be with you.
2. Ask for written instructions before you leave the doctor's office.
3. If you are not comfortable talking with your doctor, find another one. Being able to communicate with your doctor is the key to participating in your healthcare.

Chapter 2

Take Control of Your Stay in the Hospital

Objectives:

- Provide you with tips on choosing the right hospital
- Provide you with tips on staying safe in the hospital
- Provide you with tips on preventing falls and infection
- Provide you with tips on handling surgery and post-surgery care
- Provide you with on managing medications

Actual case: Taken from the *NY Times*, December 8, 2008: "Weak Oversight Lets Hospitals Stay Open" by Alex Berenson.

Sharon was admitted to University Hospital for an operation to help control her incontinence. He doctor botched her operation, causing urine to leak into her abdomen, and a second operation perforated her colon. Four years and twenty operations later, Sharon has lost most of her colon and remained incontinent. Mistakes happen at most hospitals but this particular one, which is owned by the state of New York, has had more than its fair share. In 2006 a commission recommended that it be scaled back and merged with another hospital, but the state failed to follow through. Healthgrades, a company that rates hospitals using data from Medicare, reports that University Hospital has an unusually high rate of preventable errors and ranks it among the least safe in the U.S. (see healthgrades.com).

Myth: Hospitals are the safest place to be if you are sick.

Fact: There are more than one million preventable adverse events in hospitals each year in the United States, of which 98,000 are fatal.[21] Some leading culprits are wrong site surgery, infection, medication error, and operation or post-operation complications. If you are smart and informed you can be sure you get quality, safe care. This chapter will provide you with the information you need to have a good outcome.

Finding the Right Hospital

There is no federal agency that monitors hospital quality. Use a hospital, clinic, surgery center, or other type of healthcare organization that has undergone a vigorous on-site evaluation against established state-of-the-art quality and safety standards, such as those provided by the nonprofit group the Joint Commission (jointcommision.org), which sets basic quality standards for the nation. *However, the Joint Commission lacks the enforcement powers of a regulatory agency.* They have few employees, despite accrediting and setting patient safety goals for 17,000 hospitals, nursing homes, and assisted-living providers nationwide.

> ## Do your homework before you go to the hospital.

There are Web sites available to check on your hospital's performance. Be sure your hospital is accredited by the Joint Commission by going to qualitycheck.org. The data presented on qualitynet.org comes from hospitals that *volunteered* to submit their data for public reporting in order to receive incentive pay. If your hospital did not volunteer their clinical measures, it may be wise to find another hospital. The clinical measures reported on this Web site focus on heart attack, heart failure, pneumonia, asthma (children only), and surgical care improvement/surgical infection prevention. Each rate calculation reported is based upon the hospital's relevant discharges. An acute care hospital provides inpatient medical care and other related services for surgery, acute medical conditions, or injuries (usually for a short term illness or condition). Check your area for the hospital that performs the recommended quality measures. The Hospital Quality Alliance (HQA) measure set currently consists of twenty-six measures.

A 2009 study of Medicare patients showed that patients who were treated at Distinguished Hospitals of Clinical Evidence reduced their risk of death by

---

21 "To Err is Human," Institute of Medicine, Quality of Healthcare in America, 1999.

27 percent from procedures and conditions such as cardiac surgery, angioplasty and stent, heart attack, heart failure, chronic obstructive pulmonary disease, pneumonia, stroke, abdominal aortic aneurysm repair, bowel obstruction, gastrointestinal surgeries and procedures, pancreatitis, diabetic acidosis and coma, pulmonary embolism, respiratory failure, and sepsis.[22]

This study also found that 152,666 lives may have been saved and 11,772 major complications avoided during the three years studied had the quality of care at all hospitals matched the level of those in the top 5 percent. *It is a matter of life and death—find a hospital that ranks high across all services.*[23]

To check on key treatments for which there is scientific evidence of efficacy (such as treatments for heart attack, heart failure, pneumonia, and surgical care) visit qualitycheck.org, or hospital compare.[24]

Healthgrades.com rates hospital quality in terms of mortality and complication rates across twenty-six procedures and diagnoses, from heart attacks to total knee replacement. Many hospitals excel in a given service, but very few excel across all procedures; those that do rank in the top 5 percent of hospitals and have been designated Distinguished Hospitals of Clinical Excellence.

> *Hospital death rates from three common conditions for being admitted to hospital—heart attack, heart failure, and pneumonia—can be compared by visiting hospitalcompare.hhs.gov/hospital/mortalitytool/index.asp. It is very important that you do your homework before you go to the hospital.*

Hospital Mistakes

Some hospitals have very poor safety records, as shown in Marie Lorrie Davis' recently published *How to Survive a Stay in the Hospital without Getting Killed*. For example, one in twenty patients in hospital will be given a wrong medication, and 3.5 million Americans will get an infection from someone who didn't wash their hands or take other appropriate measures. Hospitals and other medical facilities that are accredited must follow procedures to

---

22 seniorjournal.com/NEWS/Medicare/2009/20090127-MedicarePatientsReduce. htm.

23 M. L. Davis, How to Survive a Day in the Hospital Without Getting Killed, Trafford: Vancouver B.C. Canada, 2001..

24 hospitalcompare.hhs.gov/Hospital/Search/Welcome.asp?version= default&browser=IE percent7C7 percent7CWinXP&language=English&defaul tstatus=0&pagelist=Home.

avoid mistakes. Facilities that are accredited are listed on accrediting agency Web sites, such as qualitycheck.org or medicare.gov.

Adverse Medical Events ("Sentinel Events")

Adverse medical events are injuries related to medical management (in contrast to complications from a disease). Preventable adverse events are the result of errors or equipment failures—error being defined as the failure of a planned action to be completed as intended or the use of a wrong plan to achieve an aim. The Institute of Medicine estimates more than one million preventable events occur each year in the United States, resulting in between 44,000 and 98,000 deaths.[25]

The Joint Commission came up with standards to reduce medical errors,[26] however, less than one third of hospitals' reporting systems allow physicians and nurses to report errors anonymously and promise privacy for those who have identified themselves. More than 80 percent of risk managers said they had received few or no reports from physicians.[27]

The Joint Commission has identified poor communication as a root cause of adverse medical events. Rude language and hostile behavior threaten the safety and quality of healthcare.[28]

The National Quality Forum has endorsed a list of twenty-eight adverse events in hospitals for the purpose of public accountability.[29] Examples of adverse events include leaving a foreign object in a patient after surgery, operating on the wrong patient, removing the wrong body part, and falling out of bed.

Considers these other examples:

- A doctor mistakes an "a" for an "o" in a drug name.
- A doctor misplaces a decimal point in a prescription order.
- A nurse reaches for a vial in a cabinet as she has done hundreds of times before, failing to notice that the powder-blue label is more of a sky blue.

These slip-ups are often simple and always human and happen in hospitals

---

25 Kohn LT, et al. "To err is human: building a safer system. Washington D.C.: National Academy Press 2000.

26 apsf.org/resource_center/newsletter/2001/fall/08jcaho.htm.

27 ama-assn.org/amednews/2009/02/09/prse0212.htm.

28 psqh.com/enews/0708b.shtml.

29 The National Quality Forum Updates Endorsement of Serious Reportable Events in Healthcare, October 2006.

throughout the United States. In one instance, where an infant died because of a prescription error, more than fifty errors were found.[30]

Help protect yourself and your family by asking the nurse or care giver to double check that they are administering the correct medication.

The Never Event List

Medicare has been trying to force hospitals' hand in doing more to prevent adverse medical events by providing a "Never Event" list.[31] *This is a list of preventable errors for which Medicare will not reimburse hospitals.* It appears likely that private insurance companies will follow Medicare's footsteps in the near future. These errors include the following:

- Wrong surgical or other invasive procedures performed on a patient
- Surgical or other invasive procedure performed on wrong body part
- Surgical or other invasive procedure performed on the wrong patient
- Objects left in after surgery
- Air embolisms
- Blood incompatibility
- Pressure ulcers
- Falls in hospitals
- Catheter-associated urinary tract infections
- Catheter-associated vascular infections
- Mediastinitis after coronary artery bypass
- Inadequate glycemic control
- Surgical site infections
- Deep vein thrombosis and pulmonary embolism
- Drug-induced delirium

---

30 Brink S. "'It's never one thing' that leads to serious error" LA Times January 28, 2008.

31 cms.hhs.gov/apps/media/press/release.asp?Counter=1863.

What You Can Do

The Joint Commission has come up with a mnemonic to help you stay safe in the hospital: **SPEAK UP.**[32]

Speak Up
Pay attention
Educate
Advocate
Know

Use
Participate

Speak up

If you have questions or concerns and if you don't understand something ask again; it's your body and your health, so be involved. Ask yourself this question: Would you have had that procedure if you were aware of the side effects? Everything in life is risky, but by getting the information you need to make an informed decision, you mitigate the risks.

Pay attention to the care you are receiving.

Make sure you're getting the right care by the right health care professional. *Don't assume anything! Who's in charge?*[33] If you have only two doctors, they need to communicate only with you and with each other. If you have three doctors, there are six cross-paths for communication. If you have six doctors, there are potentially 720 types of doctor-doctor communication. Nobody checks that every such communication takes place and is accurate. Medical specialists often vie with each other for decision-making power. Who decides if the lung abscess needs antibiotics or surgical drainage, the lung doctors, the surgeons, or the infectious disease specialist? Just to top it off, many hospitals now employ their own *hospitalists*—primary care physicians employed by the hospital (your own primary care doctor most likely doesn't make hospital visits) who are the final decision makers at the patient's overpopulated bedside, able to overrule a specialist's and or a primary care doctor's recommendations. *You have to be your own advocate and make sure everyone involved with your care are on the same page.*

---

32 jointcommission.org/PatientSafety/SpeakUp/.
33 cancerlynx.com/10tips.html.

Educate yourself about your diagnosis, the medical tests you're undergoing, and your treatment plan.

Take an Advocate with you to the hospital to make sure you're receiving the right care and you stay safe. More about advocacy may be found in chapter 15, "The Importance of a Health Advocate."

> **I was in the hospital for an operation that required an overnight stay. At about 3:00 a.m., a nurse's aide came in to change my IV bag. Previous aides always asked my name and checked my ID bracelet. This one did not. I told her that the IV bag had been changed just one hour ago, and in fact, it was still half full. She said she was told to change Mr. Wilson's IV bag; I told her she was in Dr. Kreisberg's room! She apologized and left. Who knows what was in that bag? Good thing I'm a light sleeper!**

In conclusion, know what medications you take and why you take them. Medication errors are the most common healthcare errors. FILL OUT YOUR PILL CARD!

Use a hospital, surgery center, or other healthcare organization that has undergone a rigorous evaluation as that provided by the Joint Commission.

Participate in your healthcare; you are the center of your healthcare team.
Carry a whistle around your neck, in case you fall you can get someone's attention. Use a magic marker to mark the spot where you're supposed to be operated on.

Falls and Fall Prevention

Falls that occur in the hospital is one of the leading causes of hospital error. This is especially true for unstable elderly adults. Falls in hospitals can lead to injuries, longer stays, and higher costs. It is estimated that one million falls occur in hospitals each year![34] Medicare and many state Medicaid agencies

---

34 ahrq.gov/qual/nursehdbk/docs/Curriel_FIP.pdf.

have stopped reimbursements to hospitals for costs associated with falls, because falls are considered preventable.[35]

There are three factors that increase your likelihood of falling: intrinsic, extrinsic, and co-morbidities. *Intrinsic* factors are things that have to do with your body or how your body reacts to medication. *Extrinsic* factors are things that have to do with the hospital itself or staff. *Co-morbidities* are diseases you already have that may increase your risk of falling.

Intrinsic factors include

- Unsteady gait
- Agitation
- Epilepsy
- Increased toileting needs
- Confusion
- Sedatives or hypnotics
- History of falling
- Vitamin D deficiency
- Low PTH levels
- Anemia

Extrinsic Factors include:

- Hospital staffing
- Time of day (most falls occur during the day)
- Physical challenges (in rehab)

Co-morbidities include:

- Alzheimer's disease
- Depression
- Diabetes
- Multiple sclerosis
- Parkinson disease
- Stroke

Fall Prevention

---

35 ahrq.gov/research/dec08/1208RA4.htm.

Fall and injury screening should be performed in all settings. All patients should have comprehensive post-fall assessment done by the hospital. Ask whether your hospital performs this assessment.

See how your hospital compares to others in fall prevention by going to qualitycheck.org. Ask whether your hospital has taken action to help prevent falls. Here are some recommendations for fall intervention:

- Hospital staff is trained about safety care.
- A medical team should be trained for fall injury risk assessment and post-fall assessment.
- Hospital provides alarm devices.
- Hospital monitors medication side effects as necessary.
- Design rooms to promote safe patient movement.
- Provide exercise interventions to promote better balance.
- Provide toileting regimen for confused patients (check patients every two hours).
- Doctors monitor and treat calcium and vitamin D levels for long term care to maintain strong bones.
- Underlying disorders like diabetes and anemia, which could lead to falls, should be treated by doctors.

How to Avoid Hospital-Acquired Infections

Hospital-acquired infections kill almost one hundred thousand patients annually and account for $20 billion of healthcare costs.[36] Yet many of these infections can be avoided by following some simple guidelines. Here we present some of these guidelines you can use to help prevent some of the most common infections while in the hospital.

The first and most important thing is to make sure everyone involved with your care washes their hands before touching you. If you notice they have not, *remind them to do so*!

MRSA

Methicillin-resistant *Staphlococcus aureus* (MRSA). "Staph" is a very common germ carried on your skin. The germ does not cause problems for most people, but sometimes serious infections can occur, such as skin or wound infections, pneumonia, and blood infections. Decades-long use of unnecessary use of antibiotics has resulted in strains of *Staphloccocus aureus* that are resistant

---

36 cdc.gov/ncidod/dhqp/guidelines.html.

to methicillin. Antibiotics have been needlessly prescribed for colds, flu, and other viral infections that do not respond to antibiotics. There are approximately 368,000 cases of MRSA each year, and one out of five die from it. MRSA usually begins as small red bumps on the skin that resemble pimples or insect bites. These can quickly turn into painful abscesses that require surgical draining. These may also become life-threatening if they enter the bloodstream. Those who have other health conditions making them sick or have been hospitalized or reside in nursing home are at greatest risk for MRSA.

MRSA can be passed on to bed linens, bed rails, bathroom fixtures, and medical equipment. It may be spread to other people on contaminated equipment and on the hands of doctors, nurses, other healthcare providers, and visitors.

If you have MRSA, tell your healthcare providers. There are two types of MRSA, hospital-acquired and community-acquired.

Risk factors for hospital-acquired MRSA:[37]
- Current or recent hospitalization
- Residing in a long-term-care facility
- Invasive procedures
- Recent or long-term antibiotic use

Risk factors for community-acquired MRSA:[38]
- Young age—incomplete development of immune system
- Participation in contact sports
- Sharing towels and athletic equipment
- Living in crowded or unsanitary conditions
- Weakened immune system

Treatment
- Hospital staff must wash their hands before and after touching you.
- Wash your own hands frequently.
- Clean hospital rooms and medical equipment carefully.
- Make sure all lines and catheters are inserted and removed under sterile conditions. *Watch while these are inserted and be sure providers have washed their hands and are wearing gloves.*
- Isolation of patients—their visitors will wear gowns and gloves.

---

37 MRSA Infections JAMA 298: 1826, 2007.
38 ahrq.gov/research/dec08/1208RA4.htm.

- There are antibiotics which can be used to treat MRSA (e.g., vancomycin). Those who develop abscesses may have to have surgery to drain them.
- Hospitals should test patients for MRSA on their skin.

Clostridium Difficile Colitis[39]

Clostridium difficile colitis is a result of unnecessary use of antibiotics that disrupt or remove normal healthy bacteria from the colon. *C. diff* is identified by testing stool for the bacterium.

Risk factors
- Treatment with antibiotics
- Hospitalization
- Nursing home residency
- Critical illness
- Over sixty-five years old
- Diseases of the colon such as inflammatory bowel disease
- Recent gastrointestinal surgery

Signs and Symptoms
- Diarrhea
- Fever
- Abdominal pain or cramping
- Nausea without vomiting
- Weight loss

Treatment
- Hand washing and disinfection
- Isolation of infected patient
- Appropriate antibiotic use

Surgical Site Infections

Signs and symptoms
o Occurs at the site around the area you had surgery.

Treatment
o Most can be treated with antibiotics.

Prevention
o To prevent surgical site infections, healthcare providers

---

39 *Clostridium difficile* Colitis JAMA 301: 988, 2009

must clean their hands and arms up to their elbows with an antiseptic agent just before surgery.
- o *Clean hands with soap and water or an alcohol-based rub before and after caring for each patient.*
- o *Be sure a razor is not used to remove hair from the surgery site. Use electric clippers.*
- o Wear special hair covers, masks, gowns, and gloves during surgery to keep surgery area clean.
- o Remove hair covers, foot covers, and gowns after surgery. Never wear these items outside the operating room.
- o Give you antibiotics before the surgery begins and stop them twenty-four hours after the surgery is over.
- o Clean the skin at the site of your surgery with a special soap that kills germs.

Catheter-associated Urinary Tract Infection

A urinary catheter is a thin tube placed in the bladder through the urethra to drain urine.

A urinary tract infection is an infection of the urinary system that includes the bladder and the kidneys with germs that do not normally live in these areas.

Signs and Symptoms
- o Burning or abdominal pain, fever, or an increase in frequency of urination.

Treatment
- o Urinary tract infections can be treated with antibiotics.

Prevention
- o *Urinary tract infections can be prevented by proper catheter care—healthcare providers washing their hands before and after touching your catheter.*
- o If you go home with a urinary catheter, be sure you understand all the instructions given to you about taking care of the catheter.

Catheter-associated Bloodstream Infections

A central line or central catheter is a tube placed into a patient's large vein, usually in the neck, chest, arm, or groin. The catheter is used to draw blood or give fluids or medications. It may be left in for several weeks. A bloodstream infection develops when germs travel down the central line and enter the blood.

Signs and Symptoms
    o   If you develop an infection you will have symptoms such as soreness or redness at the catheter insertion site or fever. Immediately call your nurse or doctor if you believe you have an infection.

Treatment
    o   These infections may be serious, but often can be successfully treated with antibiotics.

Prevention
    o   Ask your doctor why you need a catheter and how long will need it.
    o   *Make sure your healthcare providers wash their hands before touching your catheter.*
    o   If you leave the hospital with a catheter, make sure you understand all instructions on how to care for the catheter.

When You Have Surgery

Pre-Surgery Routine

WHAT TO BRING WITH YOU TO THE HOSPITAL
- Your insurance/Medicare identification card
- Your Pill Card (list of medications)
- A few dollars to purchase items such as newspapers, magazines

DO NOT BRING
- Anything of value—leave your jewelry at home
- Electric razor or hair dryer

- Be sure the ID bracelet they give you is accurate!
- Tell your doctor about other medical problems you may have. Health problems such as diabetes, allergies, and obesity could affect your surgery and your treatment.

- Before you're admitted, ask your doctor if there are any medications you should avoid before your surgery. Ask whether if you should skip breakfast before coming to the hospital.
- Also, have someone take you to and from the hospital.

Once you arrive, for your safety, the staff may repeat the following questions many times:

- Who you are?
- What kind of surgery you are having?
- What part of your body is being operated on?

   o Speak up if someone tries to shave you with a razor (you do not want cuts that can become infected). They should use clippers instead. Ask why you need to be shaved and talk to your surgeon if you have any concerns. Ask if you will get antibiotics before and after your surgery. You should.

While you are awake, make sure a health professional marks the right spot on your body to operate on. Wrong-site surgery is the leading cause of unanticipated events resulting in serious injury or death (a "sentinel event"), accounting for 13 percent of such events.[40]

Ask your surgeon if he will take time out before and after your surgery to go through the checklist of standard safety procedures to double-check whether the right patient is on the operating table and the right body part to be operated on is identified. Also, at the end of surgery, they should count to make sure all the sponges and instruments are accounted for. Miscounting sponges and instruments occurs 13 percent of the time. [41]

After Your Surgery

---

40 "To Err is Human" Institute of Medicine, Quality of Healthcare in America, 1999.
41 ahrq.gov/research/jan09/0109RA17.htm.

SPEAK UP and tell your doctor or nurse about your pain. Hospitals and other surgical facilities accredited by the Joint Commission must help relieve your pain. Pain changes over time or your pain medication may not be working. Don't be a hero and suck it up; discuss your pain. Doctors and nurses should be asking about your pain regularly. There are other ways to relieve your pain. Some people use acupuncture, while others take their mind off their pain by watching movies or playing games. Sometimes, electrical nerve stimulation works to block pain and so does physical therapy, hypnosis, and massage therapy. Ask your healthcare provider for some suggestions on non-medical ways to relieve pain.

1. If you are given new medication, ask questions:

-   What is it?
-   What is it for?
-   Are there any side effects?
-   Will they interact with medications I am already taking?
-   Do you have allergies? Tell the staff about any allergies you may have.

2. What medicines will you need to take at home?
3. Get a written list of all your medications—new and old (use the Pill Card). Take this list with you to follow-up appointments. Ask questions:

-   Can you please explain the instructions that come with this medication?
-   Are there any medications or dietary supplements I should avoid?
-   What are the side effects of the medication?

4. Find out about any IV fluids you are given.
5. Ask your doctor if you will need therapy or medicines after you leave the hospital. You must leave the hospital with specific instructions to be sure you continue with the care you need for a full recovery.
6. Ask whether your primary care doctor will receive discharge instructions from the hospital.
7. Ask when you can resume activities like work, exercise, and travel.

After Your Hospital Stay

Be sure you get written instructions. Only 30 percent of patients receive them on discharge from the hospital. The written instructions should tell you how to care for your wound. Make sure you understand them. Ask your nurse whether there is someone in the hospital who could help you plan your follow-up care. The instructions should also tell you who to contact if you have questions or problems after you get home. If you have any symptoms of an infection—such as redness and pain at the surgery site, drainage, or fever—call your doctor immediately.

Other things you need to do:

- Fill any prescriptions and take all your medications.
- Ask a family member or friend to help plan your follow-up care.
- Always wash your hands before and after caring for your wound.
- If you are overwhelmed by the follow-up care, ask your nurse for a list of referrals for home care services or a skilled nursing facility.
- Find out about payment options, including whether financial assistance is available.
- Find out if the service or organization is accredited by the Joint Commission on qualitycheck.org.

Questions to ask about your condition once the procedure is completed:

- When will your doctor get a status report about your condition?
- How soon should you start feeling better?
- When you will be able to resume daily activities?
- Are there any special instructions for daily activities?
- Do you need someone to help you twenty-four hours a day?
- What signs and symptoms should you watch for and what should you do if you have any?
- Will you need any special equipment at home?
- Will you need physical therapy?
- Will you need follow-up tests?
- Who should you follow up with to get the test done?
- Will you need to schedule any follow-up visit with your doctor?
- When can you go back to work?

- Who can you call if you have any problems?

Keep Your Child Safe in the Hospital

What we discussed about your safety in the hospital also applies to your child. However, you must be your child's advocate and be sure you ask the questions listed above on their behalf. First, upon admission, be sure the information on his or her identification bracelet is correct and a bracelet is worn alerting staff to any allergies.

Here are some tips to lower the chance that your child will be harmed by his or her treatment:[42]

- Be sure anyone examining your child washes their hands before touching your child.
- Before a procedure, ask the healthcare team members whether they know exactly what the procedure is.
- Review the medications your child is taking and any other information about their care with their nurses and doctors.
- Keep an eye on all catheters and incisions, looking for evidence of infection—swelling and redness.
- Ask for a pediatrician to be involved in your child's care and whether your child should be moved to a children's hospital.
- Carry a list of all medications they are currently using.
- Always double check on the medications being prescribed and double-check that they calculated the right dose.
- READ! READ! READ! All the information you can about the medications prescribed for your child.
- Be especially vigilant if your child is taking multiple medications or high-risk medications (such as chemotherapeutic drugs, insulin, or heparin) or if your child has a compromised immune system.

To address the safety problems, Congress approved the Patient Safety and Quality Improvement Act of 2005.[43] The Patient Safety Act was approved to spur the development of voluntary, provider-driven initiatives to improve the quality, safety, and outcomes of patient care. The act, which is implemented by Agency for Healthcare Research and Quality (AHRQ) and Health and Human Services Office for Civil Rights, addresses many of the current barriers to improving patient care. All too often, healthcare

---

42 Tarkin L. "Overdoses and other medical mistakes put young patients at risk" NY Times September 15, 2008.

43 ahrq.gov/qual/psoact.htm.

providers fear that if they participate in the analysis of medical errors or patient care processes, the findings may be used against them in court or harm their professional reputations. The reluctance of providers to participate in improvement initiatives, combined with the difficulty of aggregating and sharing data confidentially across facilities or state lines, limits our current ability to aggregate data in sufficient numbers to identify rapidly the most prevalent risks and hazards in the delivery of patient care, their underlying causes, and effective practices in mitigating them.

The Patient Safety Act[44] addresses these barriers to improvement through the following goals and mechanisms:

- Encourage greater healthcare provider participation in improvement initiatives by establishing strong, nationally uniform confidentiality, and privilege protections for the patient safety information that these initiatives assemble or develop.
- Expand the analytic expertise that is available to healthcare providers to analyze safety and quality issues by encouraging the formation of new patient safety organizations (PSOs) with which providers can voluntarily work.
- Improve the ability to rapidly recognize and address the underlying causes of risks and hazards to patient care by facilitating the aggregation and analysis of large numbers of patient safety events.
- The Patient Safety Act directs the Secretary to develop regional and national statistics and trends for reporting in future AHQRs. AHRQ will carry out these activities on behalf of the Secretary and is required to develop this information through the aggregation and analysis of non-identifiable patient safety data that PSOs, providers, and others voluntarily contribute to a network of patient safety databases that the statute envisions.

---

44 ahrq.gov/qual/psoact.htm.

Chapter 3

Take Control of Your Medications

For Young and Middle-Aged Adults and Children

The Food and Drug Administration estimates that 1.3 million people suffer injuries each year and 365 die each day as a result of prescription errors. Any drug, whether it's over-the-counter or a prescription medication, has the potential to cause serious harm, even if it's used properly. This chapter will give you the information you need to protect you and your family from suffering from medication errors. Seniors have their own special concerns when it comes to medications, and these are discussed in chapter 5, section 2.

Objectives:
- To provide you with the information you need to take your medications and dietary supplements safely
- To remind you about drug abuse
- To provide you with the information you need to safely give your children medications

Actual case: Actor Dennis Quaid's newborn twins, Thomas Boone and Zoe Grace, were accidentally given a massive dose of Heparin, an anti-coagulant. Babies typically get 10 units. They were each mistakenly given the adult strength of **10,000** units. Heparin is used to flush out IV lines and prevent blood clots. Both babies started to "bleed out" and both nearly died. That same year, three babies died of the same error in a hospital in Indianapolis. There was no reason that the adult Heparin should have been stored in the neonatal ICU. It is likely that a technician picked up the wrong Heparin because both the minor dose and the major dose came in bottles that were the same color. But the similarities between the packaging of the two doses do not end there. This was easily preventable. *Since a medical error in administration could lead to a dangerous or fatal result, the vials should have been completely distinguishable in size and shape.* Prescription errors are a real enough danger in hospitals without having radically different doses of a drug being packaged in practically identical containers. Patient histories can be misread, handwriting can be hard to read, and drugs that do completely different things to the body can have practically identical names. There are simple, common-sense courses of action that pharmaceutical companies can take to at least trim the numbers a bit. Making their packaging obvious is one of them.

Because of the prevalence of prescription errors, the United States Department of Health and Human Services has come up with a system to help address this: the Pill Card, which allows you to list the medications and dosages you are taking. It fits in your wallet and is available when you go to the doctor or hospital. An example of a Pill Card may be found in the appendix.

Review your drugs with your doctor, including over-the-counter drugs, dietary supplements, and alcohol consumption. Dietary supplements include vitamins, minerals, amino acids, herbs or botanicals, and enzyme supplements. Tell your doctor about any allergies you have, including to medications such as antibiotics. Be sure to fill all your prescriptions and refills.

Be sure to provide accurate information and check what you are given at the pharmacy.

You also need to ask yourself if the pharmacy has the information they need to be sure you're safely taking you drugs. Be sure they have an accurate list of all your medications (with correct dosages), including both prescription and non-prescription drugs and supplements. The pharmacist may not ask you whether the list is accurate or not, so it's up to you to provide them the information.

Generic Drugs

Ask your doctor or pharmacist whether there are equivalent generics that may be prescribed. Generic drugs are carefully regulated medications that have the same medicinal ingredients as the original brand name drug but are generally cheaper in price. Nearly one in three drugs dispensed are generic. These undergo comparative testing to ensure that they are equal to their brand counterparts in

- *Active ingredient.* For example, "pravastatin" is the active ingredient in brand name Pravachol.
- *Dosage.* For example, 10 mg of the active ingredient.
- *Safety.* For example, same or similar side effects, drug interactions.
- *Strength.*
- *Quality.* For example, 10 mg of a generic drug can be substituted for 10 mg of the brand name and have the same therapeutic result.
- *Intended use.* For example, both generic and brand-name drug would be prescribed for the same conditions.

Off-label Use

When physicians prescribe drugs to treat certain diseases despite a lack of FDA approval, this is referred to as off-label prescribing. One out of every five prescriptions written today is for off-label use.[45] Off-label prescribing is a legal, common practice that is being questioned in some cases because of inadequate scientific evidence to support its safety and effectiveness. A new study suggests that drugs prescribed off-label for conditions for which they're not approved is *most pressing* for the medications on the following list: [46]

---

45 ahrq.gov/consumer/cc/cc042109.htm.
46 eurekalert.org/images/release_graphics/pdf/off-label-chart.pdf.

Table 3.1 Medications that are potentially dangerous when prescribed off-label

Drug (brand name)	Most-common on-label use	Most frequent off-label use
1. Quetiapine (Seroquel)	Schizophrenia	Maintenance therapy of bipolar disorder
2. Warfarin (Coumadin)	Atrial fibrillation	Hypertensive heart disease
3. Escitalopram (Lexapro)	Depression	Bipolar disorder
4. Risperidone (Risperdal)	Schizophrenia	Maintenance therapy of bipolar disorder
5. Montelukast (Singulair)	Asthma	Chronic obstructive pulmonary disease
6. Bupropion (Wellbutrin)	Depression	Bipolar disorder
7. Sertraline (Zoloft)	Depression	Bipolar disorder
8. Venlafaxine (Effexor)	Depression	Bipolar disorder
9. Celecoxib (Celebrex)	Joint sprain-strain	Fibromatosis
10. Lisinopril (Prinivil, Zestril)	Hypertension	Coronary artery disease
11. Duloxetine (Cymbalta)	Depression	Anxiety
12. Trazodone (Desyrel)	Depression	Sleep disturbance
13. Olanzapine (Zyprexa)	Schizophrenia	Depression
14. Epoetin alfa (Procrit)	Chronic renal failure	Anemia from chronic disease

Here are some questions you might want to ask your doctor concerning off-label drugs:

- Is this the approved use of the medicine? You may not know if the use is off label. This question can help you start the conversation with your doctor about your medicines.
- Is the off-label use of this drug likely to be more effective than one approved to treat my illness? This is important, because the off-label drug may not be as well tested for your condition.

- What evidence shows that this off-label drug can treat my condition?
- What are the risks and benefits of off-label treatment with this drug?
- Will my health insurance cover off-label treatment with this drug?

Picking Up a Prescription

To stay safe, ask the pharmacist the following questions when you pick up your medications.[47]

- When you pick up your prescription at the pharmacy, look at the label on the bottle to be sure you have the medication that was prescribed for you. Read the prescription label before you leave the pharmacy. Be aware that many drugs sound or look alike, such as Klonopin (a sedative) and Clonidine (for high blood pressure); oxycontin (for pain) and oxybutynin (bladder drug); colchicine (for gout) and Clonidine. *For your safety, be sure you have the correct drug.*
- Beware of different doses of the same drug in the same-looking vial.
- Carefully read the instructions or talk to the pharmacist about the following:
  - When and how do I take my medications?
  - Must I finish them, or can I stop when I'm feeling better?
  - Do I take it before, during, or after meals?
  - Does taking them three times a day mean during waking hours or over twenty-four hours?
  - Can the medication be crushed or swallowed whole?
  - Are there medications, foods, beverages, and activities to avoid, and will anything I'm taking now interact with this drug or supplement?
  - What if I miss a dose or take too much?
  - When should I seek help if symptoms persist?
  - Can I take my medicines with beverages other than water?
  - Can special needs be addressed, such as larger type of lettering on the label?
  - Are child-safe bottles available?
  - Will my over-the-counter medications interact with my prescription medications? Popular medications such as Sominex, Prilosec OTC, and Zantac have been known to do so.

---

47 Consumers Report June 2008.

Prescription Drug Abuse

Prescription drug abuse is on the rise in the United States. According to the 2003 National Survey on Drug Use and Health, 6.3 million Americans aged twelve and older have used prescription medications for non-medical purposes in the prior thirty days. In fact, prescription drugs have replaced illicit street drugs as the nation's drug of choice.[48]

- 4.7 million people used pain relievers
- 1.8 million people used tranquilizers
- 1.2 million people used stimulants
- 300,000 people used sedatives

The most frequent types of drugs abused are opioids (e.g., oxycontin, fentanyl), central nervous system depressants (valium, Xanax), and stimulants (Adderall, Ritallin).

Beware of prescription drugs mysteriously disappearing from your medicine cabinet. For twelve- to seventeen-year-olds, prescription drugs are easier to get than street drugs. They get the drugs from friends and relatives or steal them. Many get the drugs from theirs or a friend's medicine cabinet.

> **Pain killers and sedatives are now the recreational drugs of choice for teenagers and elderly adults.**

Children and Drugs

Make sure your child is safe—be your child's advocate. Unless otherwise specified, children are defined as being less than eighteen years of age.

A new study reveals that more and more children are at risk because of mix-ups in medications. The study says that about 7 percent of children being hospitalized in United States were getting wrong drugs, accidental overdoses, and unfavorable reactions.[49]

> **Surprisingly, many drugs prescribed for children have not been tested in children.**

---

48 keystonetreatment.com/oxycontin.ph.
49 vitabeat.com/adverse-drug-events-harms-us-children/v/8265/.

Only 20 percent to 30 percent of drugs approved by the Food and Drug Administration are labeled "for pediatric use." So by necessity, doctors have routinely given drugs to children off-label, which means the drug hasn't been studied in children in adequate, well-controlled clinical trials approved by the FDA. Parents must be informed about the medications their children are taking by asking the right questions.

You know your child best. If you notice something wrong after taking a medication call 911 immediately or, if they're in the hospital, get a nurse or doctor. *The doses of many medications must be adjusted based on a child's weight, and sometimes errors occur (see Quaid debacle at the start of this chapter).*

To lower the chance that your child will be harmed by a drug:

- Be sure the child's hospital identification bracelet warns of any allergies to medications.
- Prepare a Pill Card for your child and tell the doctor about any allergies your child might have.
- Familiarize yourself with the medications your child is taking so you recognize a wrong pill or liquid.
- Be watchful if your child is taking multiple medications or is on high-risk medications like chemotherapy drugs, insulin, or heparin, or if your child has a compromised immune system or organ function.

Drugs of Special Concern for Children

There are specific drugs—some of them as common as aspirin—that should not be used in children.

- Risperdal has been approved for use in children ages thirteen to seventeen with schizophrenia and for short-term use in children ages ten to seventeen with bipolar disorder.
- Children should not be treated with Serevent and Foradil for asthma. *However, never stop taking any medications without first talking to your doctor.*
- Children should not be treated with antipsychotics such as Zyprexa for behavioral disorders.
- The FDA has recommended not giving cold medications to children under two years of age.[50] Check with your pediatrician before giving your child pediatric cold medications.

---

50 ismp.org/Newsletters/ambulatory/archives/200702_1.asp.

- Children under the age of eighteen should not be given aspirin because of a potentially life-threatening disease called Reye's syndrome.
- Acetaminophen is generally considered safe in children over two months old, but you should check with your doctor for dosing instructions.
- Ibuprofen is generally safe for children over six months old, but you should check with your doctor for dosing instructions.

Vaccinations

Be sure your child gets the vaccinations he or she needs. Many parents are not having their children vaccinated because they fear it may cause autism. Many studies have looked at whether there is a relationship between vaccines and autism. The weight of the evidence indicates that vaccines are not associated with autism.[51] However, the Centers for Disease Control and Prevention (CDC) know that some parents and others may still have concerns about this issue. The CDC is committed to protecting the health of children and to identifying the biological and environmental causes of autism and other developmental disabilities, and they will continue to study the role of vaccines.[52]

Be sure that your children get the vaccinations and booster shots they need:

- Chicken pox
- DTP (diphtheria, tetanus, and pertussis)
- H. influenza B (childhood)
- Influenza
- Hepatitis A
- Hepatitis B
- MMR (measles, mumps, and rubella)
- Meningitis
- Pneumococcal (childhood)
- Polio (paralytic)
- HPV—the three-dose vaccine is routinely recommended for eleven- and twelve-year-old girls. The vaccine series can be started at nine years of age. Catch-up vaccination is recommended for thirteen-through twenty-six-year-old females who have not yet received or completed the vaccination series.[53]

---

51 cdc.gov/vaccinesafety/concerns/thimerosal.htm.
52 cdc.gov/ncbddd/autism/documents/vaccine_studies.pdf.
53 cdc.gov/std/HPV/STDFact-HPV-vaccine-hcp.htm.

Check with your pediatrician for the vaccination schedule. Childhood vaccinations not only reduce disease but are also associated with reduced healthcare costs.

Drug Interactions

The effect a drug has on you may be different from expected because that drug interacts with either another drug you're taking (drug-drug interactions), food, beverages, supplements (drug-alcohol and drug-nutrient interactions), or another disease you may have (drug-disease interactions). The effects of drug interactions may be harmful, and such interactions may increase or decrease the actions of one or more drugs, resulting in side effects or failed treatment. [54]

Drug-drug Interactions [55]

Opposing (antagonism): β-blockers such as propranolol (used to treat hypertension and high blood pressure) can counteract the effect of β adrenergic stimulants such as albuterol (taken for asthma). Non-steroidal anti-inflammatory drugs such as ibuprofen (for pain) may cause the body to retain salt and fluid and will oppose the effect of diuretics such as furosemide (for blood pressure).

Duplication effects: This can happen to people who take an over-the-counter cold medication and a sleep aid that both contain diphenhydramine or a cold remedy and pain reliever that both contain acetaminophen. Also, this can occur to people taking an opiod for pain along with *acetaminophen*.

Alteration of effect: erythromycin and ciprofloxacin decrease the enzymes that metabolize warfarin and can result in increased bleeding.

Drug-alcohol Interactions

Myth: Beer is less intoxicating than other alcoholic beverages.
Fact: One 12 oz can of beer, one 4 oz glass of wine, and one mixed cocktail are equally intoxicating.

Approximately 70 percent of Americans consume alcohol occasionally, while three in ten drink weekly.[56] With the current data on medication

---

54 merck.com/mmhe/sec02/ch013/ch013c.html.

55 merck.com/mmhe/sec02/ch013/ch013c.html.

56 pr-inside.com/three-in-ten-americans-drink-alcohol-r1252607.htm.

use (14 billion prescriptions written annually), it is inevitable that alcohol and drugs are mixed. It is estimated that adverse alcohol-drug interactions are responsible for about 25 percent of all emergency room visits.[57,58] Some specific classes of *drugs that can interact with alcohol* with dire consequences, including death, are:

- anesthetics
- antibiotics
- anticoagulants
- antidepressants
- anti-diabetic medications
- antihistamines
- anti-seizure
- anti-ulcer
- cardiovascular medication
- narcotic and non-narcotic pain medications
- sleeping pills

For a detailed discussion of drug-alcohol interactions see alcoholism. about.com/cs/alerts/l/blnaa27.htm.

Alcohol ingestion could adversely affect the actions of medications. As commented by the director of the National Institute of Alcohol Abuse and Alcoholism, Dr. Enoch Gordis,[59] "Individuals who drink alcoholic beverages should be aware that simultaneous use of alcohol and medications—both prescribed and over-the-counter—has the potential to cause problems." For example, even very small doses of alcohol probably should not be used with antihistamines and other medications with sedative effects. Individuals who drink larger amounts of alcohol may run into problems when commonly used medications (e.g., acetaminophen) are taken at the same time or even shortly after drinking has stopped. *The elderly should be especially careful of these potential problems due to their generally greater reliance on multiple medications and age-related changes in physiology.*

57 alcoholism.about.com/cs/alerts/l/blnaa27.htm.
58 gallup.com/poll/12790/Americans-Alcohol-Drink-Drank-Drunk.aspx.
59 pubs.niaaa.nih.gov/publications/aa27.htm.

Drug-nutrient Interactions

Many people do not realize that certain foods can interact with drugs and alter the effectiveness of the drugs. [60]

Table 3.2 Drug-food interactions

Affected drug	Interacting food	Interaction
Fosamax	Any food	Take with water at least ½ hr before food
Anticoagulants	Foods high in vitamin K, such as broccoli, Brussels sprouts, spinach, kale	Reduce effectiveness of drug
Certain benzodiazepines, calcium channel blockers, cyclosporine, oral contraceptives, statins	Grapefruit juice	Inhibits enzyme involved in breaking down drug resulting in increased concentration in blood
Digoxin	Oatmeal	Fiber can bind and inhibit absorption
Tetracycline	Calcium or foods containing calcium	Reduce absorption of drug

Source: Global RPh[3]

Beneficial Effects of Foods and Beverages

There are many reports of the beneficial effects of foods and beverages. For example, eating broccoli or drinking a glass of wine may boost a body's defense against cancer.[61] Salmon is a particularly good source of omega-3 fatty acids, which are known to lower LDL cholesterol while raising the good (HDL) kind.[62] Speak to your doctor about foods that can help reduce your risk of disease.

---

60 globalrph.com/drugfoodrxn.htm.
61 webmd.com/food-recipes/news/20050711/new-insight-on-how-food-helps-us-fight-cancer.
62 sixwise.com/newsletters/05/11/09/10_top_foods_to_help_you_fight_high_cho-lesterol.htm.

Drug-disease Interactions[63,64]

Table 3.3 Drug-disease interactions

Disease	Drugs	Possible adverse effects
Incontinence	β-blockers, benzodiazepines, anticholinergics, long-acting benzodiazepines, tricyclic antidepressants	Polyuria
Obesity	Zyprexa	Increased appetite, dizziness, falls, weight gain
Osteopenia	Corticosteroids	Fractures
Parkinson's disease	Antipsychotics (conventional)	Exacerbations of symptoms
Prostate disease	Non steroidal inflammatory drugs, a agonists	Urinary retention
COPD	Long-acting benzodiazepines, propranolol	CNS adverse effects, respiratory depression
Dementia	Symmetrel, psychotic drugs, muscle relaxants, anticonvulsants	Increased agitation, delirium
Falls	Benzodiazepines, tricyclic antidepressants	Increased risk of falls
Diabetes	Diuretics	Hyperglycemia

Source: Fick et al.[3]; Merck[4]

Dietary supplements are not regulated by the FDA, and there are no guarantees they contain what the label says or are not contaminated with potentially toxic chemicals and drugs. For example, it has been reported that as many as 25 percent of popular dietary supplements in the United States are contaminated with low levels of steroids and 11 percent of supplements are

---

63 Fick DM, et al: Arch Internal Medicine 163:2716-2724,2003.
64 merck.com/mmhe/sec02/ch013/ch013c.html.

contaminated with stimulants, most commonly ephedrine.[65] There are dietary supplement-drug interactions that you should be aware of.[66] That is why it's important to tell your doctor everything you are taking.

Below are some examples of dietary supplements that could be harmful.

- Ginko and anticlotting drugs (warfarin, aspirin, nonsteroid anti-inflammatory drugs) can lead to excessive bleeding.
- Echinacea, if taken for more than eight weeks, can damage the liver. If taken with other drugs, such as anabolic steroids, the risk of liver damage increases.

In conclusion, medications can be dangerous and must be used with caution. If you watch any television, you'll notice that half the commercials are advertising drugs, and they scare you half to death with all the potential side-effects. If you don't tell your doctor about the medications and supplements you're taking, as well as your alcohol and recreational drug use, you are in danger of having a serious adverse event. Remember, all drugs have side effects, and you and your doctor must weigh the risks with the benefits associated with the drugs.

---

65 steroidreport.com/2007/12/06/steroids-found-in-popular-dietary-supplements/.
66 merck.com/mmpe/sec22/ch331/ch331a.html#CIHEDIII.

Chapter 4

Take Control of Your Health Insurance

Objectives
- To gain an understanding of the different types of health insurance plans
- To help you pick the plan that's right for you and your family
- To understand your rights as the insured
- To understand the choices you have if you're uninsured or under-insured

Healthcare reform has certainly been a hot topic since the presidential campaign of 2008. By the time you read this book, healthcare reform, including affordable health insurance for everyone, will most likely be in effect. However, at the time of this writing, 48 million people were without health insurance, which means they essentially did not have access to healthcare. This section will provide you with information on how to choose an insurance plan that's right for you. Unlike citizens in most other countries, in America you need a job to have health insurance. Most Americans are provided health insurance as a benefit through their employer at group rates that are typically less expensive than individual rates. This leaves many Americans, including children, the unemployed, those who work in small businesses, and sole proprietors left to purchase individual policies that are often more expensive and require screening for health complications. However, before you begin your search on insurance companies, check the insurance regulations in your state. For example, depending on where you live, you could have access to group insurance even as a sole proprietor, which means access to insurance without being screened for health complications. To link to your state's insurance department, go to the National Association of Insurance Commissioners Web site, naic.org/state.web.htm.

Actual case: As reported by Julie Appleby in *USA Today*, September 5, 2007:

When Steve bought health insurance his agent told him the most he would have to pay out of pocket for healthcare costs would be $10,000 to $15,000 a year. It wasn't until Steve's wife found out she had cancer that he learned the policy's payment caps of $800 a night for hospital care and $1250 a day for chemotherapy were far below what each care costs. By the time his wife passed away, Steve owed more than $200,000 to hospitals and doctors. Steve was deceived; however, he bears some responsibility in that he didn't carefully read his policy or ask the right questions about exactly what was covered in his policy.

Know the Different Types of Health Insurance Plans

There are many different types of health insurance plans. Many people have a form of commercial insurance, but there are also plans for employees of the federal government, military, seniors, and children.

Commercial Health Plans

- *Health Management Organizations (HMO)* are managed care plans that require you to go to the plans' doctors and hospitals, except in medical emergency.
- *Preferred Provider Organizations (PPO)* are managed care plans that allow you to choose specialists without referral.
- *Private Fee-for-Service (PFFS)* plans allow you to go to any doctor or hospital that accepts their terms. Not all providers accept to the terms, and providers can reject or accept plans on a visit-to-visit basis.
- *Special Needs Plans (SNP)* are only for people who live in long-term care facilities or have certain illnesses.
- *Consumer-Directed Health Plans/High Deductible Health Plans (CDHP/HDHP)* are high-deductible plans with low premiums. As health savings accounts become more prevalent, there has been a shift towards HDHP. Advocates of this plan believe that shifting the

costs to the consumer will make them more cost conscious, which would exert pressure on healthcare providers to improve efficiency and quality of care. However, it now appears that consumer-directed plans actually resulted in a shift of costs from employer to employee, which doesn't decrease healthcare costs. As a result, patients put off care because they rapidly deplete their health savings accounts and are left with high out-of-pocket expenses.

Plans with a Specific Eligibility

- *Federal Employee Program (FEP)*, for employees of the federal government.[67]
- *Tricare*, for military personnel and their dependents.[68]
- MEDICARE[69] is discussed in chapter 5, "Take Control of Your Health: For Seniors."
- MEDICAID[70] is a joint federal and state program that provides healthcare coverage for income limited families with children. Income requirements change every year, so it's important to check with your state's health and human services center. Other groups of people covered by Medicaid may include people over sixty-five, the blind, the disabled, women who are pregnant, and children under nineteen (U.S. citizens and legal immigrants). Even within these groups, certain requirements such as income and assets must be met. For specific information about enrolling in Medicaid, eligibility, coverage, and services for your state, contact your local Medicaid office. You can view your state's Medicaid Office contact information by visiting the Benefits.gov Web site.

Plans for Children

The *State Children's Health Insurance Program (SCHIP)* offers free or low-cost health insurance to children from families who may not be eligible for Medicaid but still have limited incomes. As with Medicaid, states set their own eligibility requirements, but most states cover uninsured children under nineteen years old, for a family of four that earns $36,200 a year or less. For more information about your state's requirements, go to Benefits.gov. You

---

67 fepblue.org.
68 military.com/benefits/tricare.
69 cms.gov.
70 merck.com/mmpe/sec22/ch331/ch331a.html#CIHEDIII.

can get an application for SCHIP by going to Chipmedicaid.org or by calling 1-877-543-7669.

Ineligible groups may include:

- Children who are members of a family that is eligible for state employee insurance based on employment with a public agency
- Children who are residing in an institution for mental diseases
- Children who are eligible for Medicaid coverage

For answers to frequently asked questions go to Coverageforall.org or call 1-800-234-1317.

NOTE: Millions of qualified children remain uninsured primarily because they don't understand their state's requirements. Answers to frequently asked questions can be found at coverageforall.org or call 1-800-234-1317. Also, it is important to remember that you must re-qualify each year for SCHIP.

The Uninsured

There are approximately 48 million uninsured Americans. I have provided some useful tips on how to maintain your health insurance. It is important to do all you can to have some insurance in case of catastrophic illness. Remember, people who are not insured wind up with the least medical care and healthcare costs that are the greatest cause of bankruptcy.

The Economic Recovery and Reinvestment Act of 2009 provides funds for expanding Medicaid, CHIP, COBRA, and community health clinics to help the unemployed and those who live in underserved areas get the healthcare they deserve.[71] States have the option to add any of three new categories of eligible individuals:

- Anyone currently receiving unemployment assistance or who had received benefits that ran out. There would not be an income test (most states probably would not consider this option).
- Anyone fired from a job between September 2008 and January 2011 who met income eligibility standards set by the states. The applicant could not earn more than 200 percent of the federal poverty level ($21,660 for an individual; $44,100 for a family of four).
- Anyone who was fired and is receiving food stamps.

---

71 recovery.gov.

SCHIP covers children in families that earn too much for Medicaid but too little to pay for private health insurance.

COBRA

Under the Consolidated Omnibus Budget Reconciliation Act (COBRA), people who become unemployed can continue employer-provided health insurance for up to eighteen months, so long as they pay 105 percent of the premium cost—far too expensive for most people. COBRA is available to workers in firms with twenty or more employees.

- The Economic Recovery and Reinvestment Act calls for the federal government to pay 65 percent of the COBRA premium cost for up to nine months.
- Those eligible would include anyone who loses a job between September 1, 2008, and December 31, 2009. Also, the package would allow people fifty-five and older to retain COBRA coverage (at their own expense) until they get another job with medical coverage or become eligible for Medicare.

If COBRA is still too expensive, see if the following tips help:

- If you or someone in your family has a pre-existing condition, you can use COBRA at an individual rate and buy private insurance for the rest of the family.
- If you have children, keep yourself and spouse on COBRA and enroll your child in SCHIP.
- If COBRA is not an option, consider getting a high-deductible health plan that can be linked to a health savings account. This is a viable option if you are healthy and expect to have a job soon, or both. To pay for the out-of-pocket expenses, you are allowed by law to set aside $5950 ($3000 if you are single) in a non-taxed health savings account. This money can be rolled over year to year.

Community Health Centers

Health centers are the family doctor to 18 million people who are medically underserved, uninsured, or living with the barest minimum of insurance that does not cover preventive care. Many clinics charge a sliding scale fee based on your income and family size.[72]

Individual or Employer Plans

You can purchase plans directly from the insurance company (individual plans) or you can have health insurance through your employer.

Individual plans may be purchased insurance directly from an insurance company. [73,74] Go to Ehealthinsurance.com which contains information on more than ten thousand plans. You answer a few questions, enter your Zip code and date of birth, and the site will tell you which plans are available in your area.[75] Other useful information on different types of health insurance plans can be found at Coverageforall.com. Many of these sites also have customer reviews on the different plans.

- Special Needs Plans (SNP) are only for people who live in long-term care facilities or have certain illnesses.
- Consumer-Directed Health Plans/High Deductible Health Plans (CDHP/HDHP) are high-deductible plans with low premiums.

Each state imposes regulations on how insurance companies can do business. For more information, contact your state health insurance commission for help finding a policy that's right for you. As an example, the state of Texas has the following regulations:

- The state of Texas imposes cost limits on insurance policies.
- Insurance companies offering group insurance in the state of Texas must limit their exclusion period to twelve months for pre-existing conditions. Companies are allowed to review medical records up to six months prior to an application.
- Small businesses in the state of Texas may purchase group health plans, but self-employed individuals may not.
- For individual health plans, Texas does not impose a limit on insurance companies with regard to setting exclusion periods for coverage of pre-existing conditions.
- Genetic information is not considered a pre-existing condition, but pregnancy can be.

---

72 nachc.com.

73 ncqa.org.

74 ehealthinsurance.com.

75 L. Alderman, "A Guide for the Newly Jobless on Getting Health Coverage," *NY Times*, February 28, 2009.

- Texas insurance companies may deny coverage to those with a medical condition, but the state does offer an insurance risk pool to those that are rejected or cannot afford a policy. The Texas Health Insurance Risk Pool has no enrollment cap, but it does have a twelve-month exclusion period similar to other group plans. There is no annual limit on benefits, although there is a lifetime benefit cap of $1,000,000. It is likely that your state has something similar to Texas for those who have no insurance and a pre-existing condition.

Employer-Sponsored Plans

Ninety-nine percent of large companies offer health benefits for their employees and families, while 62 percent of companies with less than two hundred employees provide such benefits. Only 49 percent of small companies with two to nine employees offer health benefits. The companies that do not cite high premiums as the reason.[76]

When plans are offered, they are typically HMOs, PPOs, or PFFS plans.

Choosing a Plan

Before you choose a plan, you have to understand common insurance terms.[77,78]

- An insurance *premium* is a fee you and/or your employee pay to your insurance company to purchase a health insurance plan. These can be paid monthly, quarterly, or annually.
- A *deductible* is the amount that you must pay for covered services in a specified time period in accordance with your plan before the plan will pay benefits. The higher the deductible the lower the premiums.
- A *co-payment* is the specified dollar amount or percentage required to be paid by you or on your behalf in connection with benefits.
- *Out-of-pocket* costs include premiums, co-payments, deductibles, co-insurance, or other fees that you are required to pay outside of your health benefits plan.

---

76 californiahealthline.org/Articles/2008/9/25/Premiums-on-the-Rise-for-Employ-er-Based-Health-Insurance-Plans.aspx.

77 planforyourhealth.com/about/insurance101/.

3 dol.gov/ebsa/publications/10working4you.html.

- *Capitation* is an amount of money that an insurance company pays to a medical care provider for promised care of all the insurance company's policy holders in return.

There are coverage limits involved in most insurance plans. The majority of coverage limits deals with how much of a service the company will pay for. Once the company pays for the amount agreed upon, the policy holder will then have to pay the remainder of the bill.

There are limits for the policy holder too. They are called *out of pocket maximums*. Once the policy holder reaches the maximum amount of money paid out of his or her pocket for services, the insurance company has to pay the remainder of the bill.

And perhaps most important are *in-network providers*. These are pre-selected healthcare providers on a list of providers put together by the insurance company. These in-network providers provide medical care for a discounted price per a pre-arranged agreement with the insurance company. *Use of an out-of-network provider may not be covered by your insurance plan.*

Many insurance companies require *referrals* from your primary care doctor before you can see a specialist; otherwise, they won't pay for their services.

There are several questions that are important to answer when choosing a healthcare plan:

- How affordable is the cost of care?
- How much are monthly premiums?
- How much are the deductibles? If you and your family are young and healthy you may want to consider a less expensive high-deductible plan, which will protect you against catastrophic health costs.
- Are the co-payments or co-insurance flat fees or percentages of service fees?
- What out-of-pocket expenses have to be paid before the plan begins reimbursement?
- How does the reimbursement process work?
- What is the cost of out-of-network care?
- Does the plan cover the services that you use? Such as,
    - o Doctors, hospitals, laboratories and other health care professionals in the network
    - o Out-of-network care
    - o Treatments for pre-existing medical conditions or chronic conditions
    - o Prescription drugs

- What is the quality of the health insurance plan? Research factors of the plan such as:
  - o Ratings of the plan by independent government and non-government organizations
  - o Accreditation from groups like the National Committee for Quality Assurance[79] (NCQA) or the Joint Commission on Accreditation of Healthcare Organizations[80] (JCAHO)
- Is there a wellness program?
- What are the patient complaints?
- What are the member drop-out rates for the plan?
- What experiences do other patients have with the plan?
- What are your doctor's experiences with the plan?

You must pay careful attention to your actual medical and prescription drug expenses and out-of-pocket expenses (such as co-pay and deductibles) to see which plan suits your needs.

If you have an employer-sponsored plan, during the fall enrollment period, carefully examine your health insurance choices and pick one the suits you and your family's medical needs. For a list of the best health insurance plans, see health.usnews.com/secti ons/health/health-plans/index.html.

---

79 www.ncqa.org/.
80 jointcommission.org.

Appeals

> **To avoid any surprises because of denied claims, take the time to read your insurance policy carefully before you receive a service, have a test done, or fill a prescription. Some types of care must be pre-approved by your insurance carrier in order to have them paid for by insurance.**

If you still have questions after reading the policy, call human resources and ask someone in the benefits section to explain your coverage, or call the insurance company and have a representative explain it. If your insurance company denies your claim, you have a right to appeal the decision. Before you decide to appeal, know about the insurance company's policies governing appeals. Discuss the appeal with your doctor, because he will be part of the appeal process. If he agrees he may be able to help you with the process. An enrollee or physician may submit an oral or written request for an expedited initial determination or reconsideration if the standard timeframe of up to sixty days could jeopardize the life or health of the enrollee or the enrollee's ability to regain maximum function. The plan must notify the enrollee and physician of the determination or reconsideration no later than seventy-two hours after the receipt of the request.

> **It's your insurance company, not your doctor, who makes decisions on the care that will be paid for.**

Remember, each insurance policy has exclusions. Exclusions are predetermined services that are not covered in the plan, even if your doctor recommends such services (called "denying the claim"). If you have a service performed that is excluded, you will have to pay for that service in full. Know what your exclusions are.

Appealing a Denied Health Insurance Claim

First, know your rights. Until a patient's bill of rights is passed by Congress to strengthen opportunities to have denials reconsidered by health plans, patients are responsible for knowing the rules and regulations for appealing insurance plans. Most of the common reasons for appeals are:

- Procedure determined to be medically unnecessary
- Procedure was not a contractually covered benefit
- An out of network provider was deemed unnecessary
- An administrative issue

If you have no choice but to appeal their decision, your policy will outline the appeal process, which may involve one or two levels. It is important to pay attention to any deadlines that you must meet for appealing claims. *If you miss a deadline, your appeal won't be considered.*

In addition, the policy will also outline the appeal process. For example, most consumers will first appeal to the medical insurer, which has nurses, nurse practitioners, and physicians to review the appeals. Should that effort fail, consumers can then take their case to a state regulatory agency. If you still are having difficulties consider the following:

- **Call member services.** If you can't find your policy or you've read it and still don't understand how the appeal process works, call the member services number for your health plan and get someone to walk you through the process over the phone. Also ask for an explanation of the claim denial.
- **Get details from a phone rep about information needed for appeal.**
- **Put it in writing.** Once you have a feel for the appeal process and an understanding of why your claim was rejected, gather all your documentation (copies of your policy, the rejected claim form, your medical bill, research on your medical condition that documents that the treatment should be covered, and so on). Prepare a letter that outlines your position—that the denial should be overturned because you have proof that the medical procedure is a medical necessity and not cosmetic or whatever the denial says. There are online services to help you draft an effective appeal.[81]
- **Avoid emotionality in the appeal.**
- **Cover all the bases.** For simple clerical errors, such as a wrongly coded medical procedure or an incorrectly noted medical plan identification number, you may be able to correct the information with a phone representative and get the claim resubmitted without doing an actual formal appeal.
- If your case is less straightforward and requires more negotiation, also be sure to ask your insurance company if there are any state laws that would force the insurer to provide coverage. Sometimes insurance companies "forget" that state laws may apply in certain cases.

---

81 appeallettersonline.com/.

- **Track the details and stay organized.** It may be useful to keep a journal with dates, times of phone calls, and the names of the people you spoke with. You may need this information later in the appeal process.

- **Enlist the help of professionals to make your case.** Get your doctor involved and see if your employer has retained a health advocacy organization, such as CareCounsel,[82] to help you with medical appeals.

- **Do your own research or hire an attorney to help you.** This approach helps when a health insurance provider fails to reimburse you totally for a medical procedure because the amount charged was deemed "above average" for your area. Call other doctors in your area and find out how much they would charge. If your doctor turns out to be the cheapest, document that fact and try haggling with the medical insurer to get more of the amount covered. This won't always work, but it's worth a try.

- **Go to a higher authority.** After you've exhausted all internal appeals with the medical insurer, the next step is to go to your state's regulatory agency that oversees insurance. States have set up external medical review boards to hear appeals.[83] These review boards consist of physicians who review individual cases and insurance policies to determine what coverage should have been received. Once you reach the state level, many of the same rules apply as when you appeal to your health insurer: Keep good records, do your homework, and be persistent.

Appealing an HMO's Decision

Your HMO is required to have an appeal process that gives you the opportunity to resolve disagreements about denial of covered benefits or services.[86] HMOs may deny, limit, or terminate benefits or services if they determine they are not medically necessary. Adverse utilization management (UM) makes these determinations.

Review the services covered by your HMO and the explanation of the appeal process in your evidence of coverage. You—or your doctor, acting with your consent—have the right to file an appeal of an HMO's UM determination. There are three stages of appeal.

---

82 carecounsel.net.
83 statehealthfacts.kff.org.
86 bankrate.com/brm/news/insurance/20050726a1.asp.

Stage 1

Inform the HMO, either verbally or in writing, that you disagree with the HMO's decision to deny or limit services you believe are covered and medically necessary. A different doctor at the HMO will consider your request for services. You will receive notice of whether the HMO is revising or upholding the initial decision.

Stage 2

If you are dissatisfied with the results of the Stage 1 appeal, you can request, either verbally or in writing, that the HMO have your appeal reviewed by a panel of doctors and other healthcare professionals. You will receive notice of the panel's decision.

Stage 3

If you are dissatisfied with the HMO's decision on your Stage 2 appeal, you can file an appeal with the Department of Banking and Insurance within sixty days after receiving the HMO's Stage 2 decision. You will receive the form and instructions needed to file a Stage 3 appeal from your HMO at the same time you receive the Stage 2 appeal decision. Your case will be reviewed by independent experts under contract to the state through the Independent Health Care Appeals Program (IHCAP). Decisions made by the IHCAP are binding on the HMO.

For appeals involving urgent circumstances, the HMO is required to respond within seventy-two hours in Stages 1 and 2.

Frequently there are deadlines that must be met for an appeal to be considered.

Chapter 5

Take Control of Your Health: For Seniors

Objectives:
- To provide you with the information you need to get the right care and select the right physician
- To help you safely take medication
- To help you understand Medicare and Medicaid
- To help you plan for long-term care

Much of what you will read here was already discussed in earlier chapters. However, since senior Americans might skip the earlier chapters and go directly to senior health, I thought it warranted repeating. Seniors (ages sixty-five and older) have special healthcare requirements. To address the needs of seniors, we have divided this chapter into four sections: (1) finding a doctor, (2) medication concerns for seniors, (3) Medicare, and (4) long-term care.

SECTION 1: FINDING THE RIGHT DOCTOR AND GETTING THE RIGHT CARE

If you are a senior adult, it is important to have a *primary care doctor* (trained in either general internal medicine or family medicine) who can coordinate all your care. You will most likely, at some point, be referred to specialists for your care, and one job of the primary care physician is to keep track of and coordinate your care across all specialties. There are primary care physicians who have received further training to care for seniors. Called *gerontologists*, they are specifically trained to meet the complex medical needs of the elderly and to plan and implement interventions for common geriatric syndromes, such as dementia, delirium, drug misuse, depression, falls, incontinence, pressure ulcers, and functional decline. To find a primary care doctor or gerontologist in your area, visit abms.org or healthgrades.com.

To find physicians and other healthcare professionals who participate in Medicare go to, medicare.gov/Physician/Home.asp or advocatehealth.com/system/info/library/sam/031204.html.

You want to be sure you choose the right doctor, so remember the four signs of an unsafe practice (chapter 1):

1. The doctor doesn't listen to you.
2. The doctor's technology is in the dark ages (for example, still using paper record keeping).
3. Tour doctor doesn't contact you with lab results.
4. There have been complaints by other patients.

Be prepared for your doctor's appointment. *To ensure a good outcome, your doctor must have all the information he needs to properly examine you.* This will only happen with your cooperation. Call before your appointment for instructions.

When you go, bring the following material with you:

- Lab reports, X-rays, and contact information for any specialists or other providers that are providing care for you.
- Bring a record of all the medications you are taking. Remember your Pill Card (see appendix).
- Your family medical history.

Once you are at the doctor's office, you will need to fill out the paperwork. Keep these tips in mind:

- Show up early to fill out the paperwork.
- Answer all the questions about your medical history truthfully—this could be a matter of life and death. Your medical history is protected under the HIPAA Privacy Rule, so be honest about it. The Privacy Rule absolutely prohibits healthcare providers and plans from disclosing personal health information to employers without a patient's explicit, written authorization.

> *To get the right care, participate in your care.*
> *It is important to ask the right questions.*

Diagnosis

If asking your doctor questions about your care is too intimidating, take a friend or relative with you as an advocate. To help prevent misdiagnosis, always ask,

- What is my diagnosis (the medical name for the illness I have) and what does it mean?
- What else could my condition be?
- Could more than one thing be going on to explain my symptoms?
- Is there anything is my history, physical exam, or test results that does not fit into your diagnosis?
- How serious is my diagnosis?

And, by all means, always get a **second opinion** for any elective surgery, diagnosis of cancer, or if you feel uncomfortable or uninformed about your course of treatment.

Treatment

Before consenting to any treatments or procedures, be sure you understand what is going to be done. The following is a list of questions to ask to get the information you need to make the right decision:

1. What methods of treatment are recommended?
2. Are there other treatment options? What are they?
3. What benefits would you expect from the recommended treatments and other options?
4. What are the risks or complications of the recommended treatment and the other treatment options?
5. Are there discomforts that may be caused by the treatments?
6. What methods will be used to prevent or relieve these discomforts?
7. What are the side effects of the treatment—immediate, short-term, and long-term?
8. How will having treatment affect my normal functions and everyday activities?
9. How would not having treatment affect my normal functions and everyday activities?
10. How long will treatment last?
11. How long will it be before I can go back to my normal activities?

12. How much does the treatment cost?

Make sure you understand everything that you need to know before making an informed decision and signing an informed consent.

Testing

If you are having tests done, ask the following questions so you get the most out of the tests:
1. Are there are any foods or drinks you should avoid before or after the test?
2. When will you be notified about the results of the test?
    a. Don't assume that no news is good news. Many mistakes are made because test results get lost. Most of these are caused by communication breakdown.

Prescriptions

Chapter 2 gives more information about managing medication and includes questions to ask your pharmacist. Specific information about medications can be found in section 2 of this chapter.

If you leave with a prescription, make sure your doctor wrote it for the right drug and gave you instructions on when and how to take it. Ask if you should be concerned about drug interactions with any of the medications and dietary supplements you are taking. Confirm this with the pharmacist when you pick up your medication. Make sure everyone knows if you are allergic to any medications.

Immunizations for Seniors

The CDC recommends the following vaccines for seniors:[84]
*   Tetanus-diphtheria booster: every ten years
*   Influenza: every year
*   Herpes Zoster (shingles): once after sixty years of age
*   Pneumococcal: once at sixty-five years of age

Ask your doctor if you should have any of these. Ask for the information and take the time to read it. You don't have to get the immunization the same day you get the information from your doctor.

---

84 cdc.gov/vaccines/recs/schedules/adult-schedule.htm.

SECTION 2: TAKE CONTROL OF YOUR MEDICATIONS

Myth: Seniors can safely take the same medications as younger adults.
Fact: Seniors must be prescribed lower doses of medications, because they metabolize drugs at a slower rate than younger adults.

Know the medications and dosages you are taking and for which disease they were prescribed. One way to keep this information with you at all times is to fill out and carry a Pill Card with you. An example of the Pill Card may be found in the appendix.

Review your medications with your doctor, including over-the-counter drugs, dietary supplements, alcohol consumption, and smoking. Dietary supplements include vitamins, minerals, amino acids, herbs or botanicals, and enzyme supplements. Doctors often give seniors new prescription drugs without thoroughly assessing their other medications or supplements. Ask about dangerous interactions and side effects, because disastrous consequences can result.

According to Consumer Reports on Health, "Any new health problem in an older person should be considered drug induced until proven otherwise."

Tell your doctor about any allergies you have, including medications such as antibiotics. Ask the pharmacist the right questions when you pick up your medications. Professionals estimate that 1 in 4 hospital admissions of seniors result from medication problems, including prescription drug interactions.

Only half of all senior citizens fill their prescription medications; be sure to fill all your prescriptions—and your refills.

At the Pharmacist

When you pick up your prescription at the pharmacy, check to be sure you have the medication that was prescribed for you. Ask them:
1. Do you have my prescribing history?

2. Are there equivalent generics that you can prescribe?
3. When and how do I take my medications?
4. Must I finish them, or can I stop when I'm feeling better?
5. Do I take it before, during, or after meals?
6. Does taking them three times a day mean during waking hours or over twenty-four hours?
7. Can the medication be crushed or swallowed whole?
8. Are there medications, foods, beverages, and activities to avoid, and will anything I'm taking now interact with this drug or supplement?
9. What if I miss a dose or take too much?
10. When should I seek help if symptoms persist?
11. Can I take my medicines with beverages other than water?
12. Can special needs such as larger type of lettering on the label be addressed?
13. Will my over-the-counter medications interact with my prescription medications?

Read the prescription label before you leave the pharmacy. Beware that many drugs sound or look alike, such as Klonopin (a sedative) and Clonidnne (for high blood pressure), oxycontin (for pain) and oxybutynin (bladder drug), and colchicine (for gout) and Clonidine, so for your safety, be sure you have the correct drug. Beware of different doses of the same drug in the same looking vial. Information about generic drugs is presented in chapter 2, as well as information about off-label use and drug interactions. Please review that information for seniors.

Drug Dangers for Seniors

Ten percent of drug-associated hospital admissions are due to the abuse of benzodiazepines (valium).[85] Among persons age sixty or older, 10 percent of those in the community and 40 percent of those in nursing homes fulfill criteria for alcohol abuse.[86]

Many seniors are over-medicated and should be started on the lowest concentration of the drug titrating to higher concentrations to achieve desired effect.[87]

Non-steroidal anti-inflammatory drugs (NSAID) such as naproxen and Advil are not recommended for adults age seventy-five and older with chronic,

85 Bogunovic OJ and Greenfield SF: "Use of benzodiazepines among elderly patients. Psychiatric Services 55:233, 2004.
86 ncadi.samhsa.gov/govpubs/BKD250/26d.aspx.
87 cnn.com/2008/HEALTH/conditions/05/28/ep.age.meds/index.html.

persistent pain. Long-term use of NSAID increases the risk of heart attacks or strokes, and they don't interact well with drugs used to treat heart failure.[88]

There are forty-one drugs that are potentially dangerous to senior adults and should be avoided. The list was established by Dr. Mark Beers, and an abbreviated list is presented in the table below.[89]

Table 5.1 Potentially dangerous drugs for seniors

Drugs	Side effects	Alternatives
Anti-anxiety such as Librium, valium, and Doral	Confusion, dependence, depression, falls, prolonged sedation, incontinence	Low doses of short acting benzodiazepines such as Xanax, Ativan, and Serax
Antidepressants such as Sinequan and Prozac	Constipation, sedation, urine retention, agitation, sleep disturbances	Short acting antidepressants such as Celexa, Paxil, Zoloft
Antihistamines such as Benadryl and ChlorTrimeton	Confusion, sedation, urine retention	Zyrtec, Allegra, or Claritin
High blood pressure such as Cardura and Minipress	Dangerously low blood pressure	Diuretics
Enlarged prostate—Hytrin	Incontinence	Flomax
Pain relievers such as naproxen, Daypro, Feldene, Demerol	GI bleeding, kidney damage Confusion, falls (Demerol)	Mild pain: Tylenol, Advil; severe pain: morphine
Sleeping pills such as barbiturates (Butisol, Nembutal, Seconal), Sominex, Dalmane	Confusion, dependence, excessive sedation, falls	Low doses of short-acting sleeping pills such as Sonata and Ambien

---

88 Newoldage.blogs.nytimes.com/2009/05/06/.
89 dcri.duke.edu/curtis/beers.html.

Stomach drugs such as Dulcolax and Lomotil	Worsened bowel problems (Dulcolax); Dependence, Sedation (Lomotil)	Increased intake of fiber and fluids, change in diet, Imodium AD
Hormone replacement therapy—conjugated estrogens	Heart disease	
Antipsychotics	Treating psychotic disorders	Often used to treat agitation in dementia; shown not to be beneficial and may be toxic to seniors; more on this will be discussed in chapter on Alzheimer's

Source: *Consumer Reports Health*, September 2008, "Potentially Inappropriate Medications for the Elderly According to the Revised Beers Criteria"

Drug Interactions

Adverse drug reactions in people sixty-five years and older resulted in 58,000 emergency room visits a year—twice the number of visits of the rest of the population. An *adverse drug reaction* is defined as an unexpected or dangerous reaction to a drug. Many of these are due to accidental overdoses, allergic reactions, and prescriptions for inappropriate medications. Older persons are prescribed more long-term prescriptions as well as multiple prescriptions, which could result in misuse. A large percentage of elderly adults also use over-the-counter medications and dietary supplements along with their prescription medications, which could lead to dangerous results. The average senior citizen takes more than five prescription medications a day, and the average nursing home patient is on seven medications a day.[90]

The elderly are also at risk for prescription drug abuse, where they take drugs which are not medically necessary (e.g., pain medication). Given all this, along with the changes in drug metabolism with aging, there are likely to be more adverse health consequences among this age group. Many of these cases stem from a relatively small set of drugs that require monitoring to avoid

90 UCSF Division of Geriatrics Primary Care Lecture Series May 2001.

toxic buildup.[91] Most of these drugs have been used in clinical practice for over twenty years.

The five most common drug classes noted in these events were insulin, painkillers containing opioids, anti-clotting drugs, drugs containing the antibiotic amoxicillin, and antihistamines/cold remedies. Three of them account for 58,000 emergency room visits among people over sixty-five. They are the anti-clotting drug warfarin (also known as Coumadin), the diabetes drug insulin, and the heart drug digoxin. Digoxin toxicity occurs because the dose prescribed for seniors is the same as that for younger adults, which is too high. Seniors should receive 0.125 mg/day. Sometimes there aren't alternatives to these drugs, so doctors must be sure to manage them carefully by measuring their levels in the blood and, in the case of warfarin, measuring clotting times. Also, *seniors should be started on the lowest dose of the drug.* You may want to ask your doctor whether he is prescribing the right dose for you given your age.

Drug-drug Interactions[92,93]

Opposition (antagonism): ß-blockers, such as propranolol, used to treat hypertension and high blood pressure, can counteract the effect of ß-adrenergic stimulants, such as albuterol, taken for asthma. Non steroidal anti-inflammatory drugs such as *ibuprofen* for pain may cause the body to retain salt, and fluid will oppose the effect of diuretics such as furosemide for blood pressure.

Duplication: Many people duplicate the drugs they are taking without even knowing it. If you take an over-the-counter cold medication and a sleep aid that contain both diphenhydramine or a cold remedy and pain reliever that contains acetaminophen, you are most likely taking twice the amount that you should be taking. Consult your doctor or pharmacist when you are combining cold and prescription medications.

Alteration of effect: This occurs when one drug alters the metabolism or absorption of another drug resulting in a change in the effectiveness of the second drug. For example, erythromycin and ciprofloxacin which decrease the enzymes that metabolize warfarin can result in increased bleeding. To avoid drug interactions, discuss the medications you're taking with your doctor.

---

91 webmd.com/news/20061017/bad-events-from-drugs-are-common.

92 merck.com/mmhe/sec02/ch013/ch013c.html.

93 aging-parents-and-elder-care.com/Pages/Prescription_Drugs.html.

Drug-alcohol Interactions

It is estimated that adverse alcohol-drug interactions are responsible for about 25 percent of all emergency room visits.[94] Some specific classes of drugs that can interact with alcohol with dire consequences, including death, are

- anesthetics
- antibiotics
- anticoagulants
- antidepressants
- medications for diabetes
- antihistamines
- anti-seizure
- anti-ulcer
- cardiovascular medication
- narcotic and anti-narcotic pain medications
- sleeping pills

Alcohol-Medication Interactions: A Commentary by NIAAA Director Enoch Gordis, M.D. [95]

Individuals who drink alcoholic beverages should be aware that simultaneous use of alcohol and medications—both prescribed and over-the-counter—has the potential to cause problems. For example, even very small doses of alcohol probably should not be used with antihistamines and other medications with sedative effects. Individuals who drink larger amounts of alcohol may run into problems when commonly used medications (e.g., acetaminophen) are taken at the same time or even shortly after drinking has stopped. Elderly individuals should be especially careful of these potential problems due to their generally greater reliance on multiple medications and age-related changes in physiology.

Drug–tobacco smoking Interactions[96]

Most people do not consider the risks of cigarette smoke on medications. Below is a partial list of drugs that may be altered by smoking tobacco:

---

94 alcoholism.about.com/cs/alerts/l/blnaa27.htm.
95 pubs.niaaa.nih.gov/publications/aa27.htm.
96 From Rx for Change adapted from, Zevin S and Benowitz NL. "Drug interactions with tobacco smoking" Clin Pharmacokinet 36:425,1999.

- Xanax
- Clozaril
- Luvox
- Insulin
- Zyprexa
- Tricyclic antidepressants

Drug-food Interactions

Food has the potential to interact with drugs. Food and drug interactions may make a drug less effective, cause unexpected side effects, or increase the action of certain drugs. Some food and drug interactions can even be harmful. Potential effects depend not only on the type of drug, the dosage, and the form in which the drug is taken but also a person's age, sex, weight, nutritional status, and overall health.[97] Unless specified, it is best to take medications with water rather than fruit juices. Always discuss your medications with your doctor or pharmacist.

Drug-supplement Interactions

There are dietary supplement-drug interactions that you should be aware of.[98] Below are some examples:

- Ginko and anti-clotting drugs (warfin, aspirin, nonsteroid anti-inflammatory drugs) can lead to excessive bleeding.
- Echinacea—if taken for more than eight weeks—can damage the liver; if taken with other drugs that can damage the liver, such as anabolic steroids, risk of liver damage increases. Do not take supplements without consulting your doctor.

Disease-drug Interactions

Some drugs may have adverse side effects with certain diseases. The table below lists these effects:

---

97 newsinfo.colostate.edu/files/news_item_print.asp?news_item_id=569158928.
98 merck.com/mmhe/sec02/ch019/ch019a.html#tb019_1.

Table 5.2 List of adverse effects of drugs with certain diseases

Disease	Drugs	Possible adverse effects
Incontinence	ß-blockers, benzodiazepines, anticholinergics, long-acting benzodiazepines, tricyclic antidepressants	Polyuria
Obesity	Zyprexa	Increased appetite, dizziness, falls, weight gain
Osteopenia	Corticosteroids	Fractures
Parkinson's disease	Antipsychotics (conventional)	Exacerbations of symptoms
Prostate disease	Non-steroidal inflammatory drugs, a agonists	Urinary retention
COPD	Long-acting benzodiazepines, propranolol	CNS adverse effects, respiratory depression
Dementia	Symmetrel, psychotic drugs, muscle relaxants, anticonvulsants	Increased agitation, delirium
Falls	Benzodiazepines, tricyclic antidepressants	Increased risk of falls
Diabetes	Diuretics	Hyperglycemia

Source: Fick DM, et al. *Arch Internal Medicine* 163:2716-2724, 2003. For a more inclusive list, see merck.com/mmhe/sec02/ch013/ch013c.html.

Off-Label Prescribed Drugs

Prescribing a drug for a condition it is not intended for (off-label prescribing) is a legal, common practice that is being questioned in some cases because of inadequate scientific evidence to support its safety and effectiveness. Eighty-five percent of the 725 million total prescriptions given for the 500 drugs in 2001 were either for FDA-approved indications or off-label uses with strong scientific support. However, an estimated 150 million (21 percent) prescriptions were for off-label uses, and most (73 percent, or 15 percent of total prescriptions) of those lacked scientific support. Cardiac medications (46 percent), anticonvulsants (46 percent) and medications used to treat asthma (42 percent) were the most likely to be prescribed off-label. Psychiatric drugs were highly likely to be prescribed off-label with limited or no scientific support (96 percent vs. 4 percent strong support), as were allergy medications (89 percent vs. 11 percent strong support).[99]

Table 5.3 Commonly prescribed off-label drugs

Drug (brand name)	Most-common on-label use	Most frequent off-label use
1. Quetiapine (Seroquel)	Schizophrenia	Maintenance therapy of bipolar disorder
2. Warfarin (Coumadin)	Atrial fibrillation	Hypertensive heart disease
3. Escitalopram (Lexapro)	Depression	Bipolar disorder
4. Risperidone (Risperdal)	Schizophrenia	Maintenance therapy of bipolar disorder
5. Montelukast (Singulair)	Asthma	Chronic obstructive pulmonary disease
6. Bupropion (Wellbutrin)	Depression	Bipolar disorder

99 sciencedaily.com/releases/2006/05/060513122427.htm.

7. Sertraline (Zoloft)	Depression	Bipolar disorder
8. Venlafaxine (Effexor)	Depression	Bipolar disorder
9. Celecoxib (Celebrex)	Joint sprain-strain	Fibromatosis
10. Lisinopril (Prinivil, Zestril)	Hypertension	Coronary artery disease
11. Duloxetine (Cymbalta)	Depression	Anxiety
12. Trazodone (Desyrel)	Depression	Sleep disturbance
13. Olanzapine (Zyprexa)	Schizophrenia	Depression
14. Epoetin alfa (Procrit)	Chronic renal failure	Anemia from chronic disease

If you're concerned that you may be given a drug off-label, ask your doctor whether the drug will serve a useful purpose.

SECTION 3: UNDERSTAND MEDICARE AND MEDICAID

Medicare coverage comes in four parts: Part A, Part B, Part C, and Part D. In this section, we will discuss each part and your rights as a consumer.

You must enroll in Medicare Parts A, B, and D.[100,101] The enrollment period for Medicare A and B takes place from January 1 to March 31 and goes into effect on July 1 of the year of enrollment. You must sign up for Medicare Part D (prescription drugs) beginning November 15 and ending December 31. Each year you may review your health and prescription needs and switch to a different plan.

---

100   merck.com/mmhe/sec02/ch019/ch019a.html#tb019_1.
101   cms.gov.

Who Is Covered by Medicare? [2,102]

- People age sixty-five or older, regardless of whether they get social security benefits
- People under age sixty-five with certain disabilities
- People of all ages with end-stage renal disease (permanent kidney failure requiring dialysis or a kidney transplant).

What Does Medicare Cover?

Part A: Hospital Insurance
- Inpatient hospital care
- Skilled nursing care
- Hospice care
- Home health care (with certain restrictions)
- Most people do not pay a monthly Part A premium because they or a spouse has forty or more quarters of Medicare-covered employment.
- The Part A premium is $244 per month for people having thirty to thirty-nine quarters of Medicare-covered employment.
- The Part A premium is $443 per month for people who are not otherwise eligible for premium-free hospital insurance and have less than thirty quarters of Medicare-covered employment.

Part B: Medical Insurance
- Doctors
- Services
- Outpatient hospital care
- Durable medical equipment, such as wheelchairs and hospital beds
- Additional medical services not covered by Part A
- Premium is $96.40 a month

Remember, Medicare *does not* cover long-term care in an assisted living facility or nursing home.

Part C: Medicare Supplemental Insurance ("Medigap") A Medigap policy is health insurance sold by private insurance companies to fill the "gaps" in original Medicare plan coverage. Medigap policies help pay some of the healthcare costs that the original Medicare plan doesn't cover.

---

102   "Medicare and You 2009" call 1-800-MEDICARE for a copy.

Part D: Prescription Drug Coverage

In 2003, Congress authorized a new outpatient prescription drug benefit that took effect in 2006. Beneficiaries can get Medicare drug coverage by enrolling in either a private plan that offers the Medicare drug benefit or a Medicare Advantage plan that offers drug coverage along with Medicare's other benefits.

You must enroll for Medicare Part D (prescription drugs) each fall.

Do you Need Help Paying for Prescription Drug Coverage or Prescription Drugs?

The Medicare low-income subsidy program (Extra Help) and state-sponsored pharmaceutical assistance programs provide cost sharing or Part D premium assistance. For more information, call 1-800-MEDICARE or go to the National Conference of State Legislatures.[103]

Keep track of your medications uses and costs over the year so you can pick the plan that's right for you. Visit medicare.gov, click on prescription drug coverage Medicare Prescription Drug Plan Finder to find the plan that's right for you.

Medicaid

Medicaid is a state-administered program available only to certain low-income individuals and families who fit into an eligibility group that is recognized by federal and state law. Most of your healthcare costs are covered if you have both Medicare and Medicaid.

People with Medicaid get coverage for services not covered by Medicare, such as nursing home care and home health care. To find out whether you qualify, call your state Medicaid office. To find that phone number call 1-800-MEDICARE. *Forty-nine percent of financing for long-term care in 2004 was provided by Medicaid.*[104]

How Can I Get Help Paying for Medicare?

You must have Medicare Part A (if you qualify for help, these programs can help pay these premiums).

---

103   ncsl.org/programs/health/SPAPCCoordination.htm.
104   medicare.gov/LongTermCare/Static/Home.asp.

You must be an individual with assests less than $4000 or a couple with less than $6000 in assets. Assets include things like money in a checking or savings account and stocks and bonds. Homes and cars do not count.

An individual must have a monthly income of less than $1190 and a married couple of less than $1595. Be aware that these amounts will change each year. To keep current about changes in Medicare, periodically visit Medicarenewswatch.com.

Call your State Medicaid Assistance Office for more information (for that phone number, call 1-800-MEDICARE). Get a copy of the pamphlet "Medicare and You 2009" by calling 1-800-MEDICARE, or download one at cms.hhs.gov/Partnerships/22_MY.asp.

You may qualify for home healthcare with a Medicare-certified home healthcare agency. This is paid for by Medicare Part A. Be sure the services you require meets Medicare's quality measures. To find out how agencies rate in your area, go to medicare.gov/HHCompare/Home. asp?dest=NAV|Home|About#TabTop or go to eldercarelink.com/

Know Your Rights

The Medicare, Medicaid, and SCHIP Benefits Improvement and Protection Act (BIPA) of 2000 included provisions aimed at improving the Medicare appeals process.[105] Part of these provisions mandate that all second-level appeals, also known as reconsiderations, be conducted by qualified independent contractors (QICs). If you are enrolled in the original Medicare Plan, you can file an appeal if you think Medicare should have paid for, or did not pay enough for, an item or service you received. If you file an appeal, ask your doctor or provider for any information related to the bill that might help your case.

If you are in a Medicare Advantage Plan, and you think you are being discharged from a hospital too early, you have the right to a fast-track review by the Quality Improvement Organization (QIO) in your state. You also have access to a quick QIO review when Medicare coverage of your skilled nursing facility, home health agency, or comprehensive rehabilitation facility services are about to end. Please visit this site for more information about fast-track reviews, including the service termination notices that providers will deliver and answers to FAQs (Frequently Asked Questions). See cms. hhs.gov/MMCAG.

For detailed information about the grievance, coverage determination, and appeals processes under Medicare Part D, as well as the forms you and/ or your physician should use to make or support requests under Medicare

---

105   Medicare.gov.

Part D, see the Medicare Prescription Drug Appeals and Grievances Web page on the cms.gov.[106]

Remember, under Medicare, you have the right to get all the hospital care that you need, and any follow-up care after you leave the hospital.

SECTION 4: TAKE CONTROL OF YOUR LONG-TERM CARE

Myths about Long-Term Care

Myth: My existing health insurance plan will pay for my long-term care needs.

Fact: The overwhelming majority of health insurance plans do not protect against the costs of long-term care. Examine your existing policy.

Myth: Everyone can depend on Medicaid as a safety net.

Fact: Medicaid is a federal and state program that will pay for some types of long-term care, but only after an individual meets low-income and asset-eligibility criteria.

Myth: Families end up paying very little for long-term care.

Fact: Most long-term care costs are paid for out of pocket from the private income and life savings of individuals. In addition, unpaid family caregivers provide many resources and approximately three-fourths of the long-term care needed.

Planning for Long-term Care[107]

Long-term care comprises a variety of services that include medical and non-medical care to people who have a chronic illness or disability. Long-term care helps meet health or personal needs. Most long-term care is to assist people with support services, such as activities of daily living, including dressing, bathing, and using the bathroom. Long-term care can be provided at home and in assisted living or nursing homes. It is important to remember that you may need long-term care at any age.[108]

---

106   cms.hhs.gov/MedPrescriptDrugApplGriev.
107   Centers for Medicare and Medicaid Services, go to cms.gov and download a copy of "Medicare and you 2009" or call 1-800-MEDICARE for a free copy.
108   medicare.gov/LongTermCare/Static/Home.asp.

If Medicare or Medigap do not pay for long-term care, how do you pay for it?

- Personal resources.
- Long-term care insurance. This does not replace your Medicare coverage. For information on a policy that's right for you, contact the National Association of Insurance Commissioners (NAIC) at 1-866-470-6242.
- Medicaid is for people with limited income and assets. If you qualify for Medicaid, you may be able to get help with the costs of services that help you stay at home. Some examples of these services include homemaker services, personal care, and respite care. Call 1-800-677-1116 (Eldercare locator) for more information.
- Home and community-based programs, such as Programs for All-inclusive Care (PACE), which is a Medicare and Medicaid program that allows people who would otherwise need nursing home-level care to remain in the community.

Long-term Care Resources

Organizations you can telephone:

- Call 1-800-MEDICARE. TYY (hearing impaired) should call 1-877-486-2048.
- Call your state insurance department to get more information about long-term care insurance. For that phone number, call 1-800-MEDICARE.
- For more information about policies that meet your needs, call the National Association of Insurance Commissioners at 1-866-470-6242 for a copy of "A Shopper's Guide to Long-term Care Insurance." Call 1-800-MEDICARE to see if you qualify for coverage from Medicaid.

Organizations on the Web:

- Go to Medicare.gov and select "Plan for your long-term care needs."
- Get a copy of the "Own your future planning kit" by visiting Longtermcare.gov.
- Visit Eldercare Locator at eldercare.gov (or call 1-800-677-1116) to find the Aging and Disability Resource Center in your area. Eldercare is a free public service from the U.S. Administration on Aging.
- To examine what resources are offered by your state, go to seniorresource.com/house.htm.

A more extensive list of community resources for seniors is presented later in this chapter.

Legal Directives[109,110]

While you're healthy and "on top of your game," consider having a family meeting to discuss how you would like to live out your life as you grow older. Do not wait until a crisis occurs and you can no longer participate in this discussion. There are legal documents that can be drawn to make sure your wishes about your care are recognized in the event you are not physically or mentally capable of making them known. Since laws vary from state to state, you may want to obtain the services of an elder attorney to prepare these documents.[111]

Advanced directives are legal documents that tell the doctor what kind of care you want if you are too ill or hurt to express your wishes.[1,112] Be sure to make copies of these directives for you, your doctor, your hospital, and your long-term care facility upon admission.

Death and dying are difficult but important conversations to have. Remember, doctors are trained to save lives, even when all hope may be lost. A *living will* is an advanced directive that tells how you feel about care intended to sustain life. You have the right to accept or refuse medical care. There are many issues to address, including,

- Whether you prefer the use of dialysis and breathing machines
- Whether you want to be resuscitated if breathing or heartbeat stops

---

109   medicare.gov click on long term-care and then on long-term care planning tool.
110   nia.nih.gov "There's no place like home-For growing old."
111   neca.org.
112   familydoctor.org/online/famdocen/home/pat-advocacy/endoflife/003. printerview.html.

- Whether you want tube feeding
- Whether you wish to donate your organs
- Whether you prefer to die at home or in the hospital

A *do not resuscitate* order (DNR) is another advanced directive that tells your doctor/hospital that you do not want cardiopulmonary resuscitation if you stop breathing or your heart stops beating. *Without a DNR the doctor/ hospital will do everything in their power to resuscitate you.* If you do not want to be hospitalized if something happens to you in the nursing home or assisted living facility, you must prepare and sign a *do not hospitalize* (DNH) directive; otherwise, the nursing home is obligated to send you to the hospital if you become ill. When in the ambulance, the emergency personnel will treat you.

You can always change your mind on any advanced directive at any time, as long as you are of sound mind (that is, you can think rationally and communicate clearly). To alter an advanced directive, a document must be drawn and signed in the presence of a notary. If there is no time to write such a document, you can make your wishes known verbally in front of your doctor and the family who were present when you signed the original advanced directive. A *durable power of attorney* is an advanced directive that allows you or a designate (or surrogate) to act in your best interests and make financial and legal decisions in case you are physically or mentally impaired. A *medical durable power of attorney* allows the surrogate you designated to make medical decisions in the event you are unable to do so. Be sure to give a copy of this document to the doctor, hospital, or nursing home. If there is no medical power of attorney and you are not able to make a medical decision concerning your care the state will assign someone (a guardian) to be the medical power of attorney.

If you can afford it, get long-term care insurance and get it while you're healthy. Similar to other types of insurance, the rates are considerably lower if you obtain a policy when you're healthy; the premiums will be less than if you wait until you are older. In 2004, a semi-private room in a skilled nursing home averaged $61,685 a year.

Options for Long-Term Care

There are several options for long-term care. In this section, we will discuss aging in place (living at home), independent living, skilled nursing, assisted living, and nursing homes.

Family Care Giving[113]

More than 50 million people in the USA provide care for a chronically ill, disabled, or aged family member or friend during any given year.

Aging in Place (Living at Home)
Nine out of ten Americans desire to stay in their homes to live out the rest of their lives, because of their familiar and comfortable environments, proximity to family, independence, safety and security, and convenient access to services. If you choose this option, what should you and your family do first? [114]

1. **Assess your needs.**
   * How much help can you get from your family?
   * Could you hire someone to help you for a short time each day?
   * Do you need help with cleaning, laundry, yard work, cooking, or transportation?
   * Are you able to keep track of and pay your bills?
   * Are you able to manage, refill, and take you medications?
   * Is your home a safe place to be? Can you climb the stairs? Can you get around your home without difficulty? Do you have trouble walking? Would you benefit from a walker or wheelchair?
   * Depending on your needs, will you have to hire aides to help you with daily activities of life?

Similar to a co-op, in more than one hundred communities across the country, seniors who want to stay in their homes but cannot accomplish all of the chores that are necessary have banded together with their neighbors who are equally determined to avoid being forced from their homes by dependence.[115] Residents pay yearly dues for the security of knowing that

---

113   familycaregiversonline.com/.
114   MetLife Mature Market Institute, "Caregiving in the U.S., National Alliance for Caregiving and AARP, 2004.
115   Helpguide.org.

a prescreened carpenter, chef, computer expert, or home health aide is one phone call away.

2. **What kind of help is available?**[116]
   - Non-skilled aides
   - Adult day care
   - Aging and disability resource center
   - Caregiver programs
   - Case management
   - Elder abuse prevention program
   - Emergency response systems
   - Employment services
   - Financial assistance
   - Home health services
   - Home repair
   - Home modification
   - Information and referral/assistance information services (I&R/A)
   - Legal services
   - Nutrition services
   - Personal care
   - Respite care
   - Senior housing options
   - Senior center programs
   - Telephone reassurance
   - Transportation
   - Volunteer services

In many states, background checks are not required for people who come into your home and help you. For peace of mind, hire a professional *geriatric care manager* to help you manage your loved one's care.[117] These professionals are licensed nurses or social workers who will assess your loved one's needs and recommend care with reputable agencies. Licensed home healthcare is helpful when you are home-bound or disabled. Medicare will pay 80 percent of the costs.

If a doctor prescribes care provided by skilled personnel, it includes
   - Nursing
   - Physical and occupational therapists

---

116   eldercare.gov/Eldercare.NET/Public/Home.aspx.
117   caremanager.org.

Prevent Elder Abuse

Be aware that most elder abuse cases involve nonmedical aides hired to help around the house. If you suspect you are being abused, you probably are. You should contact family or friends or call 911 for assistance.

- Abuse isn't just physical; abusive behaviors such as screaming, yelling, and insulting or swearing are just as hurtful.
- If you find yourself losing patience and becoming increasingly short tempered with an elder you are taking care of, use community services such as senior day care to have some time for yourself.
- Be sure to check references of home aides before signing a contract.
- Monitor the care your loved one is receiving
- Intervene if problems arise
- If you hire through an agency, ask whether they've done a criminal background check on employees. Many states do not require background checks.
- Keep contact and emergency information in an accessible location.

Long-distance Care Giving

Ten percent of family caregivers live more than two hours away. There are things you can do even at a distance:

- Hire a geriatric care manager to assess your loved ones' needs and help hire reputable caregivers or place your loved ones into reputable long-term care facilities.[118]
- Install emergency call/response systems:
  - In your home
  - To wear on your person
- Prepare for an emergency:
  - Keep careful medical records, including a list of all prescription and non-prescription medications and all dietary supplements. In an emergency, the hospital (or provider) may not have all the information they need to provide you with the right care.
  - Have your insurance and Medicare identification cards handy.
  - Have your doctors' names and phone numbers handy.
  - Have family members' phone numbers handy.

Fall Prevention

---

118   familycaregiversonline.com.

Falls are a leading cause of serious injury and death among elderly people in the United States, and most falls occur in the home. [119]

Patient falls in hospitals can lead to injuries, longer hospital stays, and higher costs. Further, as of October 2008, Medicare and many state Medicaid agencies will no longer reimburse hospitals for costs associated with injuries that patients incurred when they fell while hospitalized.[120] Falls are the leading cause of injury and death and the most common cause of injury and hospital admissions among adults sixty-five and older. More than one-third of adults sixty-five and older fall each year, resulting in 360,000 to 480,000 fractures and more than 15,000 deaths. Among older people who break a hip, 29 percent die within a year. The combination of a fracture with chronic disease leads to death in 75 percent of cases.[121] Falls increase with age and in community dwellers between sixty-five and eighty-five years of age; females are more likely to fall, but males are more likely to die from fall-related injuries.[122]

> **Falls are not a part of aging. They are a warning sign of bad things to come.**

Risk factors include:[123]
- Postural hypotension
- Use of anti-anxiety medications (valium) or sedative-hypnotics
- Use of four or more prescription medications
- Environmental hazards
- Muscular strength or range of motion impairments
- Inability to get out of wheelchair
- Inability to follow instructions
- Diminished cognitive (thought) processes
- Co-morbidities
  - Diabetes
  - Parkinson's disease
  - Vitamin D deficiency
  - Gait problems

The CDC offers these tips to reduce falls at home:[124]
- Monitor medications
- Provide balance training

---

119   nihseniorhealth.gov/falls/toc.html.
120   Ahrq.gov/research/dec08/1208RA4.htm.
121   healthystates.csg.org/Publications.
122   ahrq.gov/qual/nursehdbk/docs/Curriel_FIP.pdf.
123   ahrq.gov/qual/nursehdbk/docs/Curriel_FIP.pdf.
124   cdc.gov/ncipc/duip/preventadultfalls.htm.

- Provide home safety modifications
  - o   fall proof your home
  - o   remove or avoid safety hazards
  - o   improve lighting
  - o   install handrails and grab bars
  - o   move items to make them easier to reach
- Educate about how to manage risky situations[125]
- Use a cane or walker
- Wear rubber-soled shoes so you don't slip
- Walk on grass when sidewalks are slick
- Put salt or kitty litter on icy sidewalks
- Manage underlying disorders (such as vision problems, cardiac-related syncope [temporary loss of consciousness and posture], and diabetes)

The Department of Education provides a Web site, www.abledata.com that has information on more than 30,000 products designed to make life easier and safer for people with physical limitations. No computer? Call 1-800-227-0216.

Independent Living Facilities[126,127]
Among the many senior housing options available, Independent living provides the greatest versatility and freedom. Independent living for seniors refers to residence in a compact, easy-to-maintain, private apartment or house within a community of seniors. Any housing arrangement designed exclusively for seniors (generally those ages fifty-five and over; in some cases, the age requirement is sixty-two and older) may be classified as an independent living community. To qualify, seniors must

- Be healthy and be able to live independently
- Prefer to live among their peers
- Be cognitively sound and able to communicate with doctors and caregivers
- Have the financial means or be satisfied with subsidized housing

---

125   niams.nih.gov/Health_Info/Bone/Osteoporosis/Fracture/prevent_falls_ff.asp#how.

126   MetLife Mature Market Institute, "Caregiving in the U.S., National Alliance for Caregiving and AARP, 2004.

127   Helpguide.org.

- Be able to manage their home and personal needs, compared to assisted living (which is discussed below), where residents need some assistance for activities of daily living

There are numerous types of independent living facilities:

- Retirement homes
- Senior apartments
- Senior housing
- Independent living communities
- Low-income housing
- Continuing care retirement community centers (CCRC)
  - This is the *most expensive* way to age in place; it is designed to meet seniors' health and housing needs as these needs change over time. Choosing the right facility for you depends on your financial circumstances and the amount of services you require. Independent living facilities sometimes offer the following services:

- Recreational, educational, and social activities
- Communal meals
- Local transportation
- Exercise facilities and swimming pools
- Libraries
- Beauty shops
- Gardens
- Clubhouses
- Golf courses
- Tennis and shuffleboard courts

Some retirement communities help potential customers prepare their houses for sale and refer them to real estate agents trained to work with seniors. Some retirement communities offer an extended periods to pay entrance deposits while waiting for their homes to sell. Some retirement communities help customers get short-term financing to cover their down payments.

Assisted Living[128,129,130]

Myths and Facts about Assisted Living

Myth: Assisted living can provide 24/7 care for the elderly.
Fact: Assisted living provides three meals a day and socialization. By law, such institutions are not allowed to provide medical care. If your loved one needs help going to the toilet, bathing, and dressing themselves, you will either have to do it yourself or hire home aids (at $10 to $15 an hour). In the evening after dinner, your loved one will be by herself until breakfast the next morning. If she falls out of bed, no one may know until she doesn't show up for breakfast the following morning.

Myth: A for-profit facility has more money for staff and facilities and therefore provides better care.
Fact: It has been shown that not-for-profit facilities provide better care for residents because they're not worried about satisfying stock holders. For-profit facilities run their operations on bare bone staffing to increase profits.[131]

Assisted living is less expensive than nursing home care, because it does not provide 24/7 care and does not have the necessary trained personnel to provide that care. If loved your love one requires round-the-clock nursing care, it will not be provided in assisted living. To be accepted for assisted living, your loved one should be able to evacuate the premises unassisted in case of emergency.

Resident assisted living units are for those who need some assistance in activities of daily living—such as bathing, eating, grooming, and using the toilet—but who also want to experience some independence. Assisted living facilities cost between $800 and $4000 per month. They are typically studio apartments or one-bedroom apartments with scaled-down kitchens. Assisted living units may have group dining areas and common areas for social and recreational activities. Check whether the assisted living facilities in your area are licensed by your state Department of Human Services.

I want to tell you of a personal experience we had with assisted living.

---

128   eldercare.gov.
129   Assisted living federation of America, alfa.org.
130   American Association of Homes and Services for the Aging (AASHA), aahsa.org/consumer_info.
131   Charles Duhigg, "At Many Homes, More Profit and Less Nursing", The New York Times, September 23, 2007.

When Suzanne's father had a stroke, much to our surprise, he was accepted into assisted living. There was no way he could evacuate the premises unassisted; after all, he was partially paralyzed and couldn't get out of bed unassisted. The folks at assisted living said he would be fine, so despite our anxiety, we moved him into assisted living. Before long, we were paying the assisted living facility for extra services. For example, we had to hire someone to take him to the dining room for his meals, because if he didn't make it down there on his own, he would just go hungry. After breaking his orbit after falling out of bed, we placed him into a nursing home, where he received 24/7 care. Just a caution: assisted living is a less expensive option to nursing home care but only if you can truly do things independently. It will cost you if extra help is required.

Nursing Homes

Nursing or convalescent homes are also known as skilled nursing facilities, or SNFs (pronounced "sniffs"). SNFs are live-in facilities that provide medical treatment prescribed by a physician. These nursing care facilities cater to several types of patients: some patients require short-term rehab while recovering from surgery, while others require long-term nursing and medical supervision. In addition, some SNFs offer specialized care programs for Alzheimer's or other illnesses, or short-term respite care for frail or disabled persons when a family member requires a rest from providing care in the home.

Issues to consider when selecting a nursing home:

- Is it safe?
  - o Is the unit locked?
  - o How is elopement prevented?
  - o How are falls prevented?
  - o Are physical or chemical (anti-anxiety drugs) restraints ever used? Restraints have been shown to cause more injuries than they're intended to prevent. If you suspect this happening, see the facilities ombudsman to file a complaint (see below, "Resolving Disputes with Long-term Care Facilities").
- Are assistive devices are used at the facility?
  - o Do they offer dementia healthcare?
  - o What is the range of healthcare provided by the facility?

- What is the range of treatment without having to transfer to another facility (e.g., the ER)?
- How are chronic preexisting conditions managed?
  - What are the procedures for acute care?
  - What terminal care is provided?
  - Is hospice available on the unit?
- What is the knowledge and availability of the staff?
  - What kinds of staff training programs are there?
  - What percentage of nursing assistants are certified?
  - How many hours of direct nursing care does each resident receive in a twenty-four-hour period?
  - How many full time registered nurses are there per resident?
- How is the overall quality of life for the residents?
  - Do they have daily activities?
  - Are the meals tasty?
  - Do they have a choice of meals?
  - Do they have a television room?
  - Do they have a library?
- What support services do you offer?
  - Family support groups?
  - Family education programs?
  - Care counsels?
  - Is there a full time social worker?
- Have you visited the facility?
  - Did it smell clean?
  - Were the residents asleep restrained in their wheel chairs in the corridors (which may also indicate chemical restraining)?
- Were there any Medicaid beds in the facility?

To select a nursing home in your area, go to cms.hhs.gov/ CertificationandComplianc/13_FSQRS.asp. For a list of the worst nursing homes, go to cms.hhs.gov/CertificationCompliance/downloads/SFFList. pdf.

Skilled Nursing[132]

Medicare covers skilled care in a skilled nursing facility for a disease or disability for a limited time. Examples of skilled care include changing sterile dressings and physical therapy. It is given in a Medicare-certified skilled nursing facility. As required by Medicare, you must have had a qualifying hospital stay of three consecutive days. Certain skilled care services that are needed daily on a short-term basis are covered by Medicare for up to one hundred days.

Resolving Disputes with Long-Term Care Facilities

The most common grievances filed are

- o The staff doesn't respond to resident's call lights.
- o The staff is rude.
- o The food is cold or bland.
- o The facility needs repairs.
- o The staff doesn't properly give out medications.

Seek the ombudsman assigned to your long-term care facility to help resolve disputes

The ombudsman program is an advocacy program for residents of nursing homes and assisted living facilities. As a result of the Older Americans Act, The Long-Term Care Ombudsman Program was initiated to improve the quality of care in America's nursing homes and to respond to complaints about abuse and neglect of nursing home residents. It operates in every state to ensure nursing home residents are protected. Ombudsmen are responsible for making sure that nursing home problems are resolved. They work very hard to gain the residents' trust, because many residents are afraid of reporting any problems for fear of retaliation. In addition to working with nursing homes, they also work with residents of assisted living facilities, board and care homes, and other places where residents are provided long-term care. They are either volunteers or work for the state. *They are not employed by the facility.*

If you or your loved one has an unresolved issue with a long-term care facility and need assistance to get a problem corrected, there are several ways you can find an ombudsman.

---

132   helpguide.org/elder/nursing_homes_skilled_nursing_facilities.htm.

- Check for a sign posted in the long-term care facility that lists the ombudsman's office and phone number, or ask the staff for information.
- Call your local office on aging.
- Consult the National Long-Term Care Ombudsman Resource Center's Web site for a list of ombudsmen in your state.[133]

End-of-Life Care

Nobody wants to die a slow, lingering death. However, that's how many of us die. In fact, half of us die in hospitals. Tragically, one in five patients passes away in intensive care, tethered to machines, in a lot of pain, with little respect and dignity, while futile attempts are made to "save" them. Often the "d" word has not even been discussed.[134]

Some doctors find it difficult to have end-of-life conversations, because they are afraid that it will cause the patient to become depressed and give up all hope. Actually, it has been shown that most patients who have such conversations with their doctor are no more likely to become depressed than those who do not and are *less likely* to spend their final days in the hospital. They avoid costly, futile care, and their loved ones have more peace of mind when they die.[135]

Palliative Care (Comfort Care)[136]

Defined by the World Health Organization as, "an approach that improves the quality of life of patients and their families facing the problems associated with life-threatening illness through the prevention and relief of suffering by means of early identification and impeccable assessment and treatment of pain and other problems, physical, psychosocial, and spiritual."[137]

The concern expressed by patients and family over too much aggressive care at the end of life has sparked the rise of palliative care. Palliative care takes into account the preferences of the dying patient. Be sure you have the legal papers that we talked about earlier completed before you need them so your wishes can be carried out.

---

133 ltcombudsman.org/static_pages/ombudsmen.cfm.

134 Kim Painter, "The Toughest Talking Points" USA Today December 1, 2008.

135 Marchione M. "Most cancer doctors avoid saying it's the end" Associated Press 2008.

136 Teno JM and Connor SR. "Referring a patient and family to high-quality palliative care at the close of life. We have met a new personality...with this level of compassion and empathy. JAMA 301:651, 2009.

137 Lee Hancock, "Dealing with the 'D-word', The Dallas Morning News, December 14, 2008.

Your primary care doctor would be the one to refer you for palliative care. Palliative care provides the following:

- Hospital-based care at any stage of advanced or life-threatening illness.
- *The patient and family shares in the choice of care.*
- Palliative care attends to the needs of the patient and family for practical, financial, and legal assistance.
- The patient receives competent care from an interdisciplinary team that provides evidence-based symptom palliation 24/7.
- Your care is coordinated across healthcare settings and disease trajectory.
- Compassionate care treats the patient and family with dignity and respect.
- Palliative care physicians may be certified by the American Board of Hospice and Palliative Medicine, and some achieve sub-specialization in hospice and palliative medicine by the American Board of Medical Specialties.

Hospice Care[138]

Some myths about hospice care:

Myth: Hospice is a place. [139]
Fact: Hospice care usually takes place in the comfort of your home, but it can be provided in any environment in which you live, including nursing homes, assisted living facilities, and residential care facilities.

Myth: Hospice means that the patient will soon die.
Fact: Receiving hospice care does not mean giving up hope or that death is imminent. The earlier an individual receives hospice care, the more opportunity there is to stabilize his medical condition and address other needs. Some patients actually improve and may be discharged from hospice care.

As defined in "Medicare Hospice Benefits."[140] hospice is a healthcare delivery system under which the patient opts out of curative treatments for

---

138   alz.org/carefinder/careoptions/options1.asp.
139   suttervnaandhospice.org/services/services_hospicemyths.html.
140   http://www.medicare.gov/Publications/Pubs/pdf/02154.pdf.

the terminal illness. It can take place at home, in a nursing home, in assisted living facilities, in hospitals, and in free-standing inpatient units.

Patients with life-limiting illness and a likely prognosis of six months or less if the illness runs its normal course qualify for hospice care. Also, patients with a prognosis of less than one year should be educated about hospice.

A hospice team may have one nurse for thirty patients, one to two home health aides, a full-time social worker, a part-time chaplain, volunteers, a part-time medical director, and contract therapists.

Go to the National Hospice Foundation guide on choosing a hospice.[141] Here are the key differences between hospice services and hospital-based palliative care services:

- Hospice care
  - Focus on caring for patient and family or caregivers at end-of-life.
  - Patient opts out of regular Medicare coverage for terminal illness and receives services that meet his care needs across all settings of care.
- Palliative care
  - Focus is on providing expert palliative care throughout the continuum of a life-limiting illness.
  - Can be delivered concurrently with continuing curative care or life-promoting illnesses.

Most elderly patients in their last two years of life have more unnecessary intensive treatments, tests, and days of hospitalization, *accounting for 32 percent of all Medicare spending.* Studies on Medicare spending have revealed that too many Medicare patients are receiving too much care in the last two years of life.[142,143] One study, which divided the country into 306 hospital referral regions, or regional markets for healthcare, found that the cost of care differed dramatically across different regions. The patients in the higher spending areas received 60 percent more care. For example, spending in the highest regions exceeded that of the lowest by $46,000 per patient! Terminal care was also much more aggressive in the high intensity regions, with twice as many patients seeing ten or more physicians and 63 percent more experiencing

---

141   caringinfo.org/userfiles/file/pdfs/hospiceCare/hospice_care(1).pdf.

142   Wennberg JE. "Inpatient care intensity and patient's ratings of their hospital experiences." Health Affairs 28:103, 2009.

143   Wennberg JE, et al. "Tracking care the care of patients with severe chronic illness". The Dartmouth Atlas of Health Care 2008. Executive Summary-April 2008.

death in association with an intensive care episode ("high-tech" deaths). Interestingly, those receiving more care did not have better care and were less satisfied with their care than patients in the lowest spending regions.

One of the finest healthcare organizations in the country, the Mayo Clinic, has the lowest Medicare spending. The Mayo provides an organized system of care. They are a group practice that emphasizes continuous and coordinated management of patients over time and among sectors of care. In order to achieve better care coordination and reduce overuse of acute care hospital services, the Mayo Clinic must be used as a model of healthcare delivery. Primary care "medical homes" are springing up all across the country. Do not confuse "medical home" with "nursing home"; medical homes are primary-care practices that are designed to provide coordination of care. However, in order to succeed, they must have the cooperation of specialists. The Mayo Clinic has been successful because the financial incentive has been removed by employing salaried physicians.

Reducing falls among senior adults should be a top priority for healthcare professionals. Research has shown that many falls can be prevented by addressing personal risk factors (such as monitoring medications, improving balance, and correcting visual problems) and environmental risk factors (removing tripping hazards and installing safety features such as handrails).

> **Falls are the leading cause of injury deaths and the most common cause of injury and hospital admissions among adults sixty-five or older.**

Preventing cognitive decline is also important. Cognitive health refers to a combination of mental processes commonly thought of as "knowing" and includes the ability to learn new things, intuition, judgment, language, and remembering. Having a clear mind is important for all ages, but in seniors it could mean the difference between being dependent or independent. There are some conditions and behaviors that increase the risk of cognitive decline. These include diabetes, smoking, obesity, and physical inactivity. Keeping the mind sharp is also very important.

End-of-life issues share characteristics that are similar to other public health concerns, such as substantial burden, major impact on the individual and family, financial costs to individual and society, and the potential to prevent suffering associated with the dying process. We must communicate our wishes about end-of-life with family members and healthcare providers prior to the onset of a serious illness. These conversations are important if we are to protect our autonomy in unpredictable situations.

PART 2
Take Control and Manage Chronic Disease

Chapter 6

Introduction to Chronic Disease

Myth: Chronic disease is a problem for old people. I'm young. I don't have to worry about it now.

Fact: More than 75 percent of people with chronic conditions are under the age of sixty-five.[144]

These diseases just don't "pop up" in old age. They are the accumulation of decades of unhealthy habits such as poor nutrition, lack of exercise, and alcohol and tobacco use. Early intervention can prevent or delay the onset of many chronic diseases.

In 2005, 38 percent of the U.S. population had one or more conditions classified as chronic.[145] *A chronic condition is defined as one that lasted or was expected to last twelve or more months and resulted in functional limitations and/or the need for ongoing medical care.*[1] The International Classification of Diseases has classified 111 codes as meeting the criteria for chronic conditions in adults and 177 in children. In those under twenty there were no conditions that clearly predominated. One in five people reported living with one chronic condition; 10.7 percent were living with two chronic conditions; and 13.3 percent reported living with more than two chronic conditions.

Among adults, hypertension, hyperlipidemia (high blood fat), and diabetes without complications were the most prevalent, accounting for 31 percent of all reported chronic conditions. The presence of chronic disease increased with age for the non-elderly population.[146] The most dramatic increase occurred between early adulthood (ages twenty and forty-four) and midlife (forty-five to sixty-four), an increase from 32.4 percent to 63.1 percent. After age sixty-four, people were most likely to be burdened with multiple chronic diseases (45.3 percent in younger old age [sixty-five to seventy-nine] and 54.2 percent

---

144   Paez KA, Zhao L, and Hwang W. "Rising out of Pocket Spending for Chronic Conditions: A Ten Year Trend", Health Affairs 28: 15, 2009.

145   cdc.gov/reach2010.

146   CDC "The state of aging and health in America 2007."

in old-old age [eighty years of age and older]). These populations were least likely to report no chronic conditions.[3]

An increase in life expectancy (in the past century) has extended the average lifespan almost three decades, so that the average American now has a life expectancy approaching eighty. Large numbers of individuals also live well into their eighties and many into their nineties. The U.S. population aged sixty-five and over is projected to grow from 34.6 million in 1999 to 40.4 million in 2011, to 70.3 million in 2030, and to a staggering 82.0 million by 2050. Although we are living longer than ever before, the dramatic increase in life expectancy in the United States has produced a major shift in the leading cause of death in all age groups, including older adults, from infectious diseases and acute illnesses to chronic diseases and degenerative diseases.[1]

The prevalence of chronic disease, which is largely preventable, accounts for most of our healthcare costs.

In 2002, the top three causes of death in Americans sixty-five and older were heart disease (32 percent of all deaths), cancer (22 percent), and stroke (8 percent).[147] These accounted for 61 percent of all deaths in this age group. The growth in the number of older Americans will only lead to more chronic disease, which is expensive to treat unless we change our lifestyle. Three preventable behaviors—smoking, poor diet, and physical inactivity—were the root causes of almost 35 percent of U.S. deaths.[148] These are deaths due to heart disease, stroke, diabetes, and cancer.

Five percent of our population accounts for 50 percent of our healthcare costs! The elderly (age sixty-five and over), who account for approximately 13 percent of the U.S. population, consume 36 percent of total U.S. personal healthcare expenses. Similar differences among age groups are reflected in the data on the top five percent of healthcare spenders. People sixty-five to seventy-nine (9 percent of the total population) represented 29 percent of the top five percent of spenders, and people eighty years and older (about 3 percent of the population) accounted for 14 percent of the top five percent of spenders. Over half of the people in the 5 percent group had out-of-pocket expenses that exceeded 10 percent of their family income.[149]

The per-capita cost of providing healthcare for a person sixty-five years and older is three to five times greater than someone younger than sixty-five.

---

147   http://www.cdc.gov/aging/pdf/saha_2007.pdf.

148   R. Z. Goetzel, "Does Prevention or Treatment Services Save Money? The Wrong Debate," *Health Affairs* 28: 37, 2009.

149   K. A. Paez , L. Zhao, W. and Hwang, "Rising out of Pocket Spending for Chronic Conditions: A Ten Year Trend", *Health Affairs* 28: 15, 2009.

Medicare costs have risen from $37 billion in 1980 to $336 billion in 2005, with 32 percent of costs occurring in the last two years of life. The growth in the aging population is expected to result in a 25 percent increase in healthcare costs.

Adopting healthy behaviors such as eating nutritious foods, being physically active, and avoiding tobacco use can prevent or control many of the devastating effects of these diseases. One half of all deaths in the United States can be attributable to modifiable behavioral risk factors such as smoking, alcohol use, inactivity, and poor nutrition. It is no wonder that among thirty industrialized nations, the United States ranks near the bottom on most standard measures of health status. Of all deaths from chronic diseases, 23 percent have been linked to our sedentary lifestyles alone! If just one-tenth of Americans began a moderate walking program, $5.6 billion in heart disease costs could be saved (American Heart Association). Can you imagine how wonderful our nation's health would be if we could control and prevent chronic disease?

In the following chapters we will provide you with the information you need to *get smart* and *be informed* about chronic disease so you can participate in your care, which is key to a successful outcome. Chronic conditions such as heart disease, hypertension, stroke, diabetes, cancer, chronic obstructive pulmonary disease, and dementia will be discussed, as these are the leading causes of death and disability in the United States. These diseases also cause major limitations in daily living for almost one out of ten Americans, or about 25 million people. Changes in our lifestyle, health insurance benefit design, and healthcare reform should reduce chronic conditions and improve our health.

Chapter 7

Take Control of Heart Disease

Objectives:
- To define and understand the risk factors for heart disease
- To recognize the symptoms of heart disease
- To understand the actions to prevent heart disease
- To understand treatment options in heart disease

Actual Case: As reported by Gina Kolata in her 2007 article in the *N.Y. Times*, April 8, 2007, "Lessons of Heart Disease, Learned and Ignored"

Ken Smith already suffered a heart attack at age 35. At that time he carried 278 pounds on his six feet two inch frame, his blood sugar and cholesterol levels were high, and he had a strong family history of premature death from heart attacks. Despite this he went off his medications without his doctor's consent because he got into shape and lost 45 pounds. He concluded that with his improved diet and exercise he no longer needed drugs. One week before his next doctor's appointment, he suffered a massive heart attack, but miraculously survived. The most common form of heart disease is heart attack which is caused by cardiovascular disease. *The take home message from this case is don't play doctor—take all your medications until your doctor says otherwise.*

Common Myths about heart disease:

Myth: All hospitals are the same. Any hospital can properly take care of my heart disease.
Fact: Hospitals have different performance ratings. Only half the patients who suffer from heart attack receive the most effective treatment for heart attack.

Myth: Heart disease begins in adulthood.
Fact: Teenagers can already have signs of disease in their coronary arteries.

Myth: Heart disease is just a plumbing problem caused by cholesterol clogging and blocking the arteries to the heart.
Fact: Cholesterol build up is only one cause of heart disease. The others are high blood pressure, diabetes, and smoking.

Myth: If your weight is normal and your cholesterol is normal, you're safe.
Fact: Thin people with low cholesterol die of heart attacks every day. Weight and diet are only part of the story. You also need to quit smoking, exercise, and control your blood pressure and blood sugar.

Myth: Women get breast cancer, not heart disease.
Fact: Heart disease kills far more women than breast cancer. Women past the age of menopause are at particular risk.

Myth: If you take statins to control your blood cholesterol, you can eat whatever you want.
Fact: Statins can cut your risk of cardiac events. But without eating properly, exercising, not smoking, and controlling your blood pressure, you're still at risk for heart attack.

Heart Disease Defined

Heart disease is the number-one killer in the United States and a major cause of disability, as it has been for nearly a century. The most common cause of heart disease is *heart attack*. The term heart disease is often used interchangeably with "cardiovascular disease," a term that generally refers to conditions that involve narrowed or blocked blood vessels that can lead to a heart attack, chest pain (angina), or stroke. [150] Cholesterol-containing plaque builds up in the wall of the coronary arteries (a condition called atherosclerosis). Over time, the lumen of the vessel that supplies blood to the heart muscle is narrowed because of plaque buildup. The blood supply to the heart is reduced. A clot may suddenly form on top of the plaque, obstructing blood flow, resulting in a heart attack or myocardial infarction.

Cardiac arrest is the sudden loss of heart function. Without immediate cardiopulmonary resuscitation (CPR) or electrical shock of the heart (with an automated external defibrillator), there is little chance of survival: only

---

150   mayoclinic.com/health/heart-disease/DS01120.

4.6 percent of patients who suffer cardiac arrest survive. The cardiac arrest victim may or may not have been diagnosed with heart disease, but the most common cause of cardiac arrest is cardiovascular disease.

Other heart problems involve damage to the valves in the heart, high blood pressure, or improper heart pumping resulting in heart failure (congestive heart failure). *Heart failure is the most common hospital admission diagnosis in patients age sixty-five or older, accounting for more than 700,000 hospitalizations among Medicare beneficiaries every year.* Nearly 16 million Americans live with heart disease, and the most common cause of heart failure is coronary vascular disease and heart attack. There are one million heart attacks each year and 500,000 deaths.[151]

Cardiac Arrest[152]

Sudden death from cardiac arrest is a major health problem that's received much less publicity than heart attack. The American Heart Association supports implementing the "chain of survival" to rescue people who suffer a cardiac arrest in the community. The adult chain consists of the following:

- Early recognition of the emergency and activation of emergency response system (phone 9-1-1 immediately)
- Early CPR
- Early defibrillation
- Early advanced care

Sudden cardiac death results from an abrupt loss of heart function (cardiac arrest). The victim may or may not have diagnosed heart disease. The time and mode of death are *unexpected*. It occurs within minutes after symptoms appear. The most common underlying reason for patients to die suddenly from cardiac arrest is coronary vascular disease.

About 310,000 people a year die of cardiovascular disease without being hospitalized or admitted to an emergency room. That's about half of all deaths from coronary vascular disease—about 850 Americans each day. Most of these are sudden deaths caused by cardiac arrest.

Approximately 6.4 percent of out of hospital cardiac arrests victims survive to discharge. The mortality rate from sudden cardiac death has not changed over the past half century.

Brain injury is the common cause of morbidity and mortality of cardiac arrest.

---

151   mayoclinic.com/health/heart-attack/DS00094
152   ahrq.gov/clinic/uspstf/uspsacad.htm.

What Causes Sudden Cardiac Death?

All known heart diseases can lead to cardiac arrest and sudden cardiac death. Most of the cardiac arrests that lead to sudden death occur when the electrical impulses in the diseased heart become rapid (ventricular tachycardia) or chaotic (ventricular fibrillation) or both. This irregular heart rhythm (arrhythmia) causes the heart to suddenly stop beating.

In 90 percent of adult victims of sudden cardiac death, two or more major coronary arteries were narrowed by fatty buildups. Scarring from a prior heart attack is found in two thirds of victims.

When sudden death occurs in young adults, other heart abnormalities are more likely causes. Adrenaline released during intense physical or athletic activity often acts as a trigger for sudden death when these abnormalities are present. Under certain conditions, various heart medications and other drugs—as well as illegal drug abuse—can lead to abnormal heart rhythms that cause sudden death.

Can Cardiac Arrest That Causes Sudden Death Be Reversed?

Brain death begins in just four to six minutes after someone experiences cardiac arrest. Cardiac arrest is reversible in most victims if it's treated within a few minutes with an electric shock to the heart to restore a normal heartbeat. CPR can double or triple a cardiac arrest victim's chances of survival. *Few attempts at resuscitation succeed after ten minutes. If someone becomes unconscious, call 9-1-1 immediately. They may be suffering from sudden cardiac arrest.* Recently, delicate patient cooling has increased the survival of patients with cardiac arrest in coma for twelve to twenty-four hours.[153] A study published in the New England Journal of Medicine in 2002 found that 55 percent of patients that received the cooling treatment ended up with moderate or no brain damage compared with 39 percent who did not. Mortality rates were 44 percent with the cooling and 51 percent without. About half of all emergency rooms use cooling treatment.

> *If you haven't already done so,
> take a class in CPR at your
> local YMCA. It could save
> someone's life.*

---

153   *N.Y. Times*, December 4, 2008.

Risk Factors for Heart Disease

Cardiovascular disease is the number-one killer of women in the United States. Long thought of as primarily affecting men, we now know that coronary artery disease also affects a substantial number of women. Experts estimate that one in two women will die of heart disease or stroke, compared with one in twenty-five women who will die of breast cancer.[154]

From 1980 to 2000, the age-adjusted death rate for coronary artery disease fell to 266 per 100,000 men from 542 deaths and to 134 deaths per 100,000 women from 263.[155] The change meant 341,745 fewer coronary deaths in 2000 than would have otherwise occurred! The explanation for this drop is attributed to CPR, aspirin regimens, controlling diet, statin use to reduce cholesterol levels, drugs that lower blood pressure, a decline in smoking, controlling weight, a small rise in physical activity, clot dissolving medications, angioplasty, and bypass surgery. All told, nearly 168,000 deaths were preventable or delayed.[3]

> *So far, there doesn't appear to be a reversal of these trends; however, unless we do something to control the burgeoning weight gain in this country, the risk factors for heart disease will continue to increase and deaths from heart disease will rise again.*

> **It has shown that use of aspirin, beta-blockers, and clot-busters prevents future heart attacks.**

A recent two-year study on diet, published in the New England Journal of Medicine, found that it didn't matter whether the diet emphasized protein, fat, or carbohydrates; all were equally successful in promoting weight loss and maintaining weight loss over the two-year period of the study.[156] *What was important in reducing weight was eating fewer calories.* Yes, we must reduce the portion size that we consume. You can eat most anything you want; you just have to eat less of it. Weight reduction was also associated with improved cholesterol levels and less insulin resistance.

Recent statistics show significant differences between male and female survival rates following a heart attack. For example, 42 percent of women who

---

154   ahrq.gov/research/womheart.htm.

155   Brody JE. "In matters of the heart, prevention is the key" NY Times July 31, 2007.

156   F. M. Sacks et al., "Comparison of Weight Loss Diets with Different Compositions of Fat, Protein, and Carbohydrates," *NEJM* 360: 859, 2009.

have heart attacks die within one year, compared with 24 percent of men. Of those who initially survive, 23 percent of men and 31 percent of women will have another MI within six years. The reasons for these differences are not well understood. We know that women tend to get heart disease about ten years later in life than men, and they are more likely to have coexisting chronic conditions. Research also has shown that women may not be diagnosed or treated as aggressively as men, and their symptoms may be very different from those of men who are having a heart attack.[157]

Symptoms of Heart Disease

It is important to recognize the symptoms of a heart attack and recognize that women may have different symptoms than men.[158]

Typical heart attack symptoms:

- Chest discomfort or pain
- Upper body pain and pain spreads from your chest to your shoulders, arms, back, neck, teeth
- Stomach pain, which may feel like heartburn
- Shortness of breath
- Anxiety
- Lightheadedness
- Sweating

Many women *do not have chest pain* with heart attack!

Common heart attack symptoms in women include:

- Neck, upper back, shoulder, jaw, or abdominal discomfort
- Shortness of breath
- Nausea or vomiting
- Abdominal pain or heartburn
- Lightheadedness
- Unusual or unexplained fatigue

Because of these different symptoms, women are often misdiagnosed as having a gastric disorder because of vomiting or heartburn, anxiety disorder,

---

157   americanheart.org/presenter.jhtml?identifier=4632.
158   mayoclinic.com/health/heart-attack/DS00094/DSECTION=symptoms.

or chronic fatigue syndrome. If you are diagnosed with these disorders, you should ask your doctor if he has ruled out heart disease.

During a heart attack, some people waste precious minutes because they don't recognize the important signs and symptoms, or they deny them. Some people also delay calling for help because they're afraid to risk the embarrassment of a false alarm. Do not call a cab or have a friend or drive yourself to the hospital. With an ambulance, the hospital will be expecting you and be ready to treat you immediately.

> **Don't be embarrassed about being wrong or "tough it out." You are wasting precious minutes. Only 10 percent of heart attack victims get to the hospital within one hour when treatment is optional. Call 911.**

Do not go to a neighborhood urgent care center, because they often don't have the necessary equipment to treat heart attack victims!

If it turns out you weren't having a heart attack, doctors may be able to pinpoint the cause of your signs and symptoms and treat them. Plan ahead and know which hospitals in your area give state of the art care for heart disease.

Risk Factors for Heart Disease

You are considered at high risk for heart attack or coronary death if you have one or more of the following risk factors:[159]

- Family history of heart disease
- Male gender
- Cigarette smoking
- High blood cholesterol or triglycerides[160]
  - High density lipoproteins (HDL, "good" cholesterol) less than 35 mg/dL
  - Low density lipoproteins (LDL, "bad" cholesterol) greater than 130 mg/dL
  - Triglycerides 250 mg/dL or higher.

Diet as a Risk Factor
Your diet may also be a risk factor, especially if it is high in trans-fats. Trans-fats are BAD FATS, so avoid food that contain them. The American Heart

---

159   hin.nhlbi.nih.gov/atpiii/calculator.asp?usertype=prof.
160   ahrq.gov/clinic/uspstf/uspsacad.htm.

Association suggests you limit total fat intake to less than 25–35 percent of your total calories each day, limit saturated fat intake calories, and limit trans-fat intake.[161] Read the nutrition labels on all food products to see how much fat is coming from saturated fats.

The remaining fat should come from sources of monounsaturated and polyunsaturated fats such as nuts, seeds, fish, and vegetable oils. You should limit cholesterol intake especially if you have coronary artery disease or your LDL cholesterol level is 100 mg/dL or greater.

Fish oil/omega-3 fatty acids benefit the hearts of healthy people and those at high risk of cardiovascular disease. The American Heart Association makes the following recommendations for omega-3 fatty acid intake:[162]

- Patients *without* documented coronary artery disease should eat a variety of fatty fish at least two times a week. Include oils and foods rich in alpha-linolenic acid (flaxseed, canola, and soybean oils; flaxseed and walnuts).
- Patients *with* documented coronary artery disease should consume about 1 g of EPA+DHA[163] per day preferably from fatty fish. EPA+DHA in capsule form should be considered only after consulting with your physician.
- Patients who need to lower their triglycerides should take 3 to 4 g of EPA+DHA per day provided as capsules. Tell your doctor you are taking this supplement. High intake of EPA+DHA could cause excessive bleeding in some people.

In conjunction with your diet, physical activity helps prevent heart disease, because it can help prevent obesity. Obesity is defined as a body mass index, BMI, greater than or equal to 30 kg/m2. To calculate your BMI, go to nytimes.com/ref/health/bmi.html.

Hypertension (High Blood Pressure) as a Risk Factor
You have hypertension if your systolic blood pressure greater 140 mm Hg or higher or your diastolic blood pressure is 90 mm Hg or higher. Hypertension can be diagnosed only after two or more elevated readings on at least two visits over a period of one to several weeks (see following chapter on hypertension).

---

161   americanheart.org/presenter.jhtml?identifier=532.
162   americanheart.org/presenter.jhtml?identifier=4632.
163   eicosapentaenoic acid (EPA) and docosahexaenoic acid (DHA).

Other Risk Factors

Other illnesses and environmental factors present risk factors for developing heart disease:

- Diabetes
- Stress
- Alcohol
- Vitamin D deficiency increases risk of heart attack by 60 percent.[164] Vitamin D appears to have effects well beyond building healthy bones that are still unclear.
- Women who take Hormone Replacement Therapy (HRT) for just a few years during menopause have little to worry about having an increased risk of heart disease, but they should take it only to relieve symptoms and not to prevent heart disease.[165] Talk to your doctor about HRT.
- High blood levels of high sensitivity-C-Reactive Protein ($_{hs}$-CRP).

Preventing Heart Disease

Men with any of the above risk factors should be screened annually, starting at twenty-five to thirty-five years of age, for blood cholesterol, triglyceride and $_{hs}$-CRP levels. Women should be screened at thirty-five to forty-five.

If you don't have any risk factors, all men over thirty-five and women over forty-five should be screened for blood cholesterol levels, triglycerides, and $_{hs}$-CRP. To accurately measure blood cholesterol and triglyceride levels, the test requires that you have not eaten for twelve hours prior to having your blood drawn.

Screening for high blood pressure by your doctor should begin at age eighteen.[166]

Make sure you take all your medications and refill your medications that your doctors give you. *Remember you are at greater risk of suffering a second heart attack than you were for the first heart attack*. It's very important to follow your doctor's instructions.

If you've had a heart attack or have any risk factors for heart disease, your doctor may recommend taking a single baby aspirin (81 mg) daily. However, be aware that ibuprofen counteracts the effects of aspirin. If you're taking a single dose of ibuprofen, wait eight hours to take aspirin or take the ibuprofen thirty minutes after the aspirin. You should also ask your doctor about vitamin D supplements.

164   americanheart.org/presenter.jhtml?identifier=3052800.
165   webmd.com/news/20030303/timing-of-hrt-key-to-heart-benefit.
166   ahrq.gov/clinic/uspstf/uspshype.htm.

Heart Disease Treatment

Only a small fraction of the nation's acute care hospitals offer treatment such as angioplasty that can open clogged arteries. Yet many hospitals will admit patients for such procedures despite not having the expertise on hand to do it safely. To be sure your hospital is experienced in interventional cardiac procedures (they perform a large volume of them), find a designated "best" heart hospital in your area.[167]

If patients do not get the right treatment within an hour, there will be permanent damage to the heart muscle. Only 10 percent get to the hospital in time. If you think you're having a heart attack, chew one 325 mg aspirin or four baby aspirins, and tell the doctors at the hospital that you took aspirin.

The tests your doctor will perform to determine whether your signs and symptoms are the result of a heart attack are as follows:

- Electrocardiogram
- Blood tests to search for enzymes released from damaged heart muscle

If you are having a heart attack the doctors will proceed to immediately treat you.
You may have an angiogram and a possible angioplasty (placing a metal stent into a clogged artery).

Factors That Affect the Choice of Treatment in Coronary Artery Disease

Treatment of coronary artery disease depends on a number of factors, along with your personal preferences and general health status.

Stenting or bypass surgery may be used for patients in the throes of a heart attack. Several major medical associations that deal with heart disease issued new criteria for treating patients with clogged arteries. It said artery-opening procedures weren't necessary for patients with milder symptoms who weren't treated with drugs.[168]

The panel recommended surgery or stenting only after patients continued to have severe symptoms and were already taking the best available medication.[169]

---

167   jointcommission.org/CertificationPrograms/Disease-SpecificCare/
DSCOrgs.

168   news.morningstar.com/newsnet/ViewNews.aspx?article=/DJ/2009010514
15DOWJONESDJONLINE000380_univ.xml.

169   Mark DB. Quality of life after late invasive therapy for occluded arteries.
NEJM 360: 774, 2009.

Significant blockage in the left main coronary artery usually requires surgery. Bypass surgery (instead of angioplasty) may be needed.[170]

If two to three heart arteries are blocked, the type of treatment will depend on the location and severity of the blockages, how they are affecting heart function, and how severe a person's symptoms are. If only one artery is blocked (other than the left main artery), medication or angioplasty is most often used.

Be sure to ask your doctor what your treatment options are, and ask about the risks of treatment. Also be sure to ask your doctor how many times he has performed these procedures. The procedures should have been done enough times that they have become routine (literally, hundreds). Angioplasties are usually done by an interventional cardiologist and bypass surgery by a cardiovascular surgeon. For help in finding an expert, go to www.ucomparehealth.com or go to a Center of Excellence in Cardiovascular Disease in your area.

Coronary artery bypass graft (CABG) is when a section of vein from the patient's leg is removed and sewn above and below the clogged coronary artery. *If this is an elective procedure, get a second opinion.* Studies performed at Harvard and Brown medical schools showed that 10 percent of bypass surgeries performed on Medicare patients were not appropriate, and 40,000 were entirely unnecessary.

There is a 1 to 2 percent mortality rate from the surgery, and 4.5 percent suffer cognitive defects such as memory loss, confusion, or depression. This is thought to be due to being put on a heart lung machine during the surgery (known as "pump-head").

If it is necessary for you to have bypass surgery, find the best hospital in your area by going to jointcommission.org/CertificationPrograms/Disease-SpecificCare/DSCOrgs.

Best Practice Treatments for Heart Attacks[171]

You may be given the following:

- Aspirin, immediately when you arrive at the hospital, to dissolve any clots that have formed in your coronary arteries.
- Super aspirins such as Plavix.

---

170   Serruys PW. "Percutaneous coronary intervention versus coronary artery bypass grafting for severe coronary artery disease" NEJM 360: 961, 2009.

171   mayoclinic.com/health/coronary-artery-disease/DS00064/ DSECTION=treatments-and-drugs.

- Clot-busters, intravenously, to quickly dissolve clots before they damage heart muscle or cause death. If clot busters are unsuccessful, stenting or bypass surgery may be necessary.
- Pain medication to relieve discomfort.
- Nitroglycerin to temporarily open clogged vessels.
- Digoxin to increase the strengthen heart muscle contraction. If you are a senior, your doctor may give you half the normal dose (0.125 mg/day) and carefully evaluate you for potential adverse drug interactions.
- ß-blockers to help relax your heart muscle, slow your heartbeat, and decrease your blood pressure to keep your heart from working too hard.
- Angiotensin converting enzyme inhibitor (ACE) to dilate blood vessels to lower blood pressure and allow better blood flow. One possible side effect of ACE inhibitors is persistent cough. In that case, your doctor may substitute an angiotensin receptor blocker (ABR).
- Cholesterol-lowering medication, such as the statins.
- Diuretics to decrease fluid accumulation in the body.

Rehabilitation

The purpose of rehabilitation is to promote healing of your heart and prevent another heart attack. Some hospitals offer cardiac rehabilitation programs that may start while you're in the hospital and, depending on the severity of your attack, continue for weeks to months after you return home. Cardiac rehabilitation programs generally focus on three main areas—medications, lifestyle changes, and emotional issues.

It is not uncommon to feel anger, guilt, or depression following a heart attack. Talk to your family and doctor about these feelings (see chapter 14, "How Our Emotions Affect Our Health"). It is as important to take care of your psychological health as it is your physical health.

Talk to your doctor about when it is safe to resume sexual activity. Some medications may interfere with your desire for sex, but more often than not, this is psychological.

Heart disease has many components, but there are many things you can do to prevent it from happening to you. Are you eating a variety of healthy foods, exercising, and paying closer attention to portion control, managing the *amount* of food that you eat (as your total calorie intake determines your weight)? Many people have trouble losing weight and keeping weight off after they lose it. See if your employer has a wellness program that provides counselors to assist in weight loss programs or if your insurance covers weight loss programs. I would recommend staying away from any supplements that advertise weight loss. They are not regulated by the FDA and could be unsafe.

You should also control your hypertension (high blood pressure, see the next chapter) and high cholesterol. If diet or lifestyle changes do not lower your blood pressure, or high blood cholesterol and triglycerides, discuss treatment with statins with your doctor. Statins also have been shown to reduce $_{hs}$-CRP levels.

Just fifteen minutes of exercise five days a week has been shown to decrease cardiac death by 46 percent.[172] Exercise raises good cholesterol (HDL) and helps to lower bad cholesterol (LDL), and more oxygen to your muscles and tissues may help manage your weight.

Active and passive smoke and other tobacco use can raise cholesterol, damage your lungs and blood vessels, and cause cancer.

In addition, avoid artificial trans-fats; they raise LDL (bad) cholesterol and lower HDL (good) cholesterol and have been squarely linked to heart disease. New York City has even banned the use of trans-fats in restaurant cooking! Eat a diet rich in fruits, vegetables, and whole-grain products.

Tell your doctor about all the medications you're taking, including over-the-counter and dietary supplements, and tell your doctor about any side effects after starting a medication.

Finally, get the proper amount of sleep.

Don't stop taking your medications because you're feeling better! Never stop taking your medication until your doctor tells you to.

---

172   runningonline.com/zine/Health/68.sht.

Chapter 8

Take Control of Hypertension

Objectives
- Understand the risk factors of hypertension
- Recognize the symptoms of hypertension
- Know how to prevent hypertension
- Taking control of your hypertension

Actual Case: Ten years ago, a sixty-year-old female went to the doctor complaining of recurrent dizziness and headache, and her blood pressure was 170/70 mm Hg (normal being 120/80). She was given medications to control her blood pressure. However, one year ago she stopped taking her medications, because she thought her blood pressure was under control. She again visited the doctor when her symptoms returned. Further tests revealed her blood pressure was elevated, and now there was damage to her heart and kidneys. Half of all Americans older than sixty have hypertension. *Don't stop taking your meds without talking to your doctor!*

Some Common Myths about Hypertension:

Myth: Hypertension is always accompanied by symptoms.
Fact: Most often hypertension has no symptoms, which is often why it is called the "silent killer."

Myth: Hypertension affects only adults.
Fact: About 3 percent of children have hypertension, and it appears to be linked to childhood obesity.

Definitions[173]

Understanding the terms associated with hypertension is important to understanding the disease process.

a. *Systolic blood pressure* (upper number). Normal is less than 120 mm Hg.
b. *Diastolic blood pressure* (bottom number). Normal is less than 80 mm Hg.
c. *Normotensive* people have blood pressure less than 120/80 mm Hg.
d. *Hypertension.* Blood pressure is greater than 140/90 mm Hg.
e. *Prehypertension.* Blood pressure is between 120/80 and 140/90 mm Hg. Prehypertensive people have twice the risk of developing hypertension of normotensive people.
f. *Essential hypertension (primary hypertension)* has no clear cause and is thought to be linked to genetics, poor diet, lack of exercise, and obesity.[174] This is the common type of high blood.
g. *Secondary hypertension* is high blood pressure caused by other conditions that affect your kidneys, arteries, heart, or endocrine system.[175]

Risk Factors for Hypertension

There are two types of risk factors for hypertension, preventable and non-preventable.

Non-preventable

- *Age.* The chance of hypertension increases with age. Greater than fifty-five years of age for men and over sixty-five for women.
- *Race.* High blood pressure develops at an earlier in African Americans, and complications such as stroke and heart attack are more common in African Americans.
- *Family history.* Hypertension runs in families.

Preventable

- *Smoking.*
- *Obesity* (body mass index greater or equal to 30 kg/m^2).

173   mayoclinic.com/health/high-blood-pressure/DS00100.
174   mayoclinic.com/health/secondary-hypertension/DS01114.
175   mayoclinic.com/health/high-blood-pressure/DS00100.

- *Too much salt in your diet.* Read the labels on the products you buy for the amount of salt. A high sodium diet might increase the risk of hypertension and subsequent heart attack, kidney disease, and stroke. Guidelines recommend that healthy adults get no more than 2300 mg of sodium a day (*the amount in one teaspoon*). One glass of vegetable juice cocktail contains 650 mg salt. Also, remember that restaurants use salt liberally in food preparation, so ask for low-salt meals.
- *Lack of exercise.*
- *Chronic diseases* such as kidney disease and diabetes.

Symptoms of Hypertension[176]

NOTE: Hypertension usually does not cause symptoms, which is why it is necessary to be screened for hypertension. Some possible symptoms include,

---

- Severe headache
- Fatigue
- Confusion
- Blurred and double vision
- Nausea and vomiting
- Anxiety
- Perspiration
- Angina like pain (crushing chest pain)

Diagnosing Hypertension

Have your blood pressure measured and know what it is. Hypertension is the most diagnosed primary disorder in America, yet only *30 percent* are aware they have high blood pressure.[177] Blood pressure measurements should begin at eighteen years of age and must be repeated over time. People forty and older should have annual physical exams to help prevent chronic disease from developing. *Your doctor should provide you with your blood pressure measurement, in writing, as well as your blood pressure goals, if you have high blood pressure.*

If a person has had undiagnosed hypertension for a long while, a physician will assess organ damage and evidence of cardiovascular disease. What they commonly look for:

---

176   mayoclinic.com/health/high-blood-pressure/HI99999.
177   news-medical.net/news/2007/05/02/24579.aspx.

1. Enlarged heart
2. Angina or heart attack
3. Heart failure
4. Stroke or transient attack
5. Chronic kidney disease
6. Retinopathy
7. Peripheral vascular disease

Even if you have not been diagnosed with high blood pressure, it is important to have your blood pressure checked annually, especially if you have a history of high blood pressure in your family.

Treatment

If you're over sixty, there's a good chance you have hypertension.[178] *If you do not have high blood pressure at age fifty-five, you have a 90 percent chance of developing it in your lifetime.* Get an annual checkup to have your blood pressure monitored. Not treating your blood pressure increases your risk for heart attack, stroke, and kidney disease.

If you have high blood pressure, make sure you get it under control by working with your doctor on treatment goals. Only 50 percent of people with hypertension have their blood pressure under control (<140/90 mm Hg).[179]

Patients who have a co-morbid condition (such as diabetes and chronic kidney disease) along with hypertension should reduce their blood pressure to <130/80.

Most hypertensive people can get their blood pressure under control with lifestyle changes and medications. However, if your doctor doesn't discuss lifestyle changes with you or prescribe adequate medications, inadequate blood pressure control may result. It is important for you to take control of your blood pressure. In clinical trials, antihypertensive therapy resulted in a 35–40 percent reduction in strokes, a 20–25 percent reduction in heart attacks, and a 50 percent reduction in heart failure.[180]

NOTE: Pseudoephedrine hydrochloride (PH) is a decongestant that also elevates blood pressure. Many over-the-counter cold and sinus medications contain PH. For those taking medication for high blood pressure, these products are not recommended.

---

178   nhlbi.nih.gov/hbp/hbp/whathbp.htm.
179   umm.edu/features/blood_pressure.htm.
180   health.am/hypertension/more/hypertension-treatment-results-from-clini-cal-trials/.

In cases where lifestyle changes do not bring lower blood pressure, medications are used to control it. Most people need two or more such medications to control blood pressure. Some of these medications include:

- Angiotensin converting enzyme (ACE) inhibitors, such as Zestril (ACE inhibitors may cause coughing)
- Angiotensin receptor blockers (ARBs), such as Advent
- Beta-blockers such as Atenolol
- Calcium channel blockers such as Isopton
- Direct renin inhibitors, including Tekturna
- Diuretics such as Lasix
- Vasodilators such as Loniten

Essential hypertension is controllable with proper treatment. It requires lifelong monitoring, and treatment may require periodic adjustments. Pre-hypertension may be controlled by lifestyle changes (nutritional and exercise).

Hypertension affects 50 million people in the United States, and it is an independent risk factor for cardiovascular disease. Because hypertension does not cause symptoms until there is serious damage, it is important to detect it early. Hypertension is a silent killer that can lead to heart attack, heart failure, stroke, and kidney disease. The "Seventh Report of the Joint National Committee on Prevention, Detection, Evaluation, and Treatment of High Blood Pressure" provided the following new guidelines for hypertension:[181]

- In people over fifty, a systolic blood pressure over 140 mm Hg is a more important cardiovascular risk factor than diastolic blood pressure.
- Individuals with prehypertension should be counseled for healthy lifestyle modifications such as weight loss, exercise, limited alcohol intake, and nutritional changes to prevent cardiovascular.

The risk of damage to your heart and blood vessels beginning at a blood pressure of 115/75 mm Hg doubles with each increment of 20/10mm Hg. Individuals who are normotensive at fifty-five years of age have a 90 percent chance of developing hypertension sometime in their lifetime.

---

181   nhlbi.nih.gov/guidelines/hypertension/.

Chapter 9

Take Control of Stroke

Objectives:
- To understand the risk factors for stroke
- To recognize the symptoms of stroke
- To understand preventative measures
- To know what to do if you suffer a stroke and how to treat it

Actual Case Report: As reported in the *NY Times,* May 28, 2007, by Gina Kolata, "Lifesaving Opportunities Missed Before and After Stroke"

Fifty-three-year-old Dr. Jane Fowler knew her blood pressure was too high—200/120—but was convinced she was too young for blood pressure medications. On her way to work one morning, for a split second the right side of her body felt weak. Suddenly her car began to swerve. Her right food was dead, but she was able to steer her way into a parking lot. She tried to call 911 but was unable to speak. This is when she realized she had a stroke. She was lucky because she wound up at a hospital with the equipment and expertise to accurately diagnose and treat it. Most people aren't so fortunate and wind up with brain damage having to spend the rest of their lives in a nursing home.

In another example, an otherwise healthy seventy-nine-year-old man was told after an exam that he had a diseased heart valve that should be replaced. After suffering a heart attack in his forties, he quit smoking, watched his diet, and to the day of his exam vigorously exercised three times a week with no discomfort. Despite this, the doctor recommended replacing his valve while he was "healthy," to avoid complications that might take place when he developed symptoms. The night following surgery he suffered a stroke, which left him partially paralyzed and unable to care for himself. He spent the last three years of his life in assisted living and nursing homes depleting all his retirement savings. Let this be a lesson to us all—open-heart surgery is for the very sick, not for those without symptoms: *Get a second opinion if you're considering elective surgery.*

Myth: I live in America! Of course I'll get the right care if I have a stroke. All hospitals are the same.

Fact: Only 3 percent of Americans suffering from the most common type of stroke get the right care.

Stroke Defined

Stoke is the third leading cause of death in this country, accounting for 150,000 deaths. Stroke is the leading cause of serious long-term disability in the United States, costing the nation $62.7 billion a year.[182] Along the road from diagnosis to treatment to rehabilitation to stroke prevention, however, is a litany of missed opportunities.[2] A stroke may occur when an atherosclerotic plaque from a diseased coronary or carotid artery ruptures and lodges in a cerebral artery (called an *ischemic stroke*). A stroke may also occur if there is a bleed into the brain caused by a ruptured aneuryism (called a *hemorrhagic stroke*). In both cases, blood flow to the brain is interrupted. It is estimated that 1.9 million nerve cells and 7.5 miles of nerve fiber die each minute following a stroke.

As discussed by Gina Kolata in the *New York Times,* many deaths and disabilities are preventable, because either the victim does not get to the hospital in time or the emergency room they're taken to is not equipped to determine whether the only drug useful to treat stroke victims, tissue

---

182   strokecenter.org/patients/stats.htm.

plasminogen activator, is appropriate.[183] Indeed, only 3 percent of patients who could benefit from this drug are treated with it. *The key here is to be taken to a stroke center.*

Risks for Developing Stroke[184,185]

Hypertension (blood pressure greater than 140/90 mm Hg)

Even if your blood pressure is normal you should have it measured annually if you have a family history of hypertension or if you are fifty-five years of age or older. Normotensive people over the age of fifty-five have a 90 percent chance of developing hypertension. Only 30 percent of people with hypertension know they have it, and of those that do know, only 50 percent have it under control.

Your doctor should write down for you your blood pressure and blood pressure treatment goals. Be sure and take all your blood pressure medications. Once blood pressure therapy is initiated, you should have monthly monitoring until your blood pressure goals are met.

Once your goals are met, blood pressure should be measured every three months. Once your blood pressure is under control you should have semi-annual blood pressure checks and take your medications. You will be on blood pressure medications for the rest of your life.

> **Lowering your blood pressure reduces the risk of stroke 35–40 percent.**

High Cholesterol (240 mg/dL or above)

Dietary modifications and/or statin therapy are used to lower cholesterol levels. Exercising decreases your risk of stroke by elevating good cholesterol (HDL). Other lifestyle changes that lower cholesterol levels include:

- Stop smoking and using smokeless tobacco
- Drink alcohol in moderation, if at all

---

183 Gina Kolata, New York Times (May 28, 2007, "Lifesaving Opportunities Missed, Before and After Stroke."

184 stroke.org/site/PageNavigator/HOME.

185 mayoclinic.com/health/stroke/DS00150.

Diabetes

Recently, the Centers for Disease Control and Prevention reported that the number of Americans with diabetes had grown to about 24 million, with people sixty and over accounting for 25 percent of the cases. Most of the deaths from diabetes are due to the complications it causes. Diabetes increases your risk of heart disease and stroke, kidney disease, blindness, nervous system disease, periodontal disease, and amputations. It is a disease that literally can eat you from the inside out. Despite its seriousness, a recent poll showed that the public knew little about this disease and the complications associated with it.[186] Diabetes will be discussed in detail in chapter 10.

The risk for stroke is two to four times higher among people with diabetes.

Atrial Fibrillation (AF)

AF is an irregular heartbeat that changes how your heart works and allows blood to collect in the chambers of your heart. This blood, which is not moving through your body, tends to clot. The beating of your heart can move one of these blood clots into your blood stream and can cause a stroke. Your doctor can diagnose AF by carefully taking your pulse. AF can be confirmed or ruled out with an electrocardiogram (ECG) (a recording of the electrical activity of the heart), which can probably be done in your doctor's office.

If you have AF, your doctor may choose to lower your risk for stroke by prescribing medicines called blood thinners. Aspirin and warfarin are the most commonly prescribed treatments.

Previous Transient Ischemic Attacks (TIA)

This is when blood flow to the brain is transiently interrupted, so you will see some of the symptoms of stroke come and go, which could be a sign of an imminent full-blown stroke.

---

186   nytimes.com/2008/07/01/health/01iht-01well.14123321.html?_
       r=1&scp=1&sq=diabetes:%20underrated,%20insidious%20and%20
       deadly&st=cse.

Vitamin D Deficiency

Vitamin D levels below 10 ng/ml increase the risk of stroke by 62 percent. Have your blood vitamin D levels measured by measuring 25 dihydroxy vitamin D. Vitamin D levels should be greater than 30 ng/ml.

Female Hormone Replacement Therapy (HRT)

It's thought that HRT raises stroke risk by increasing the chances of formation of blood clots.[187] However, many doctors suggest that short-term use of HRT to relieve menopausal symptom—such as hot flashes and vaginal dryness—may benefit some women when it's taken at the right time. Talk to your doctor about the risks of HRT.

Symptoms and Warning Signs of Stroke[188,189]

Knowing the warning signs of stroke could be the difference between life and death. The sooner you get to the hospital, the better your chances for survival. The following are common signs of stroke:

- Sudden numbness of the face, arms, or legs, especially on one side of the body
- One side of the face droops
- Inability to raise both arms
- Sudden trouble walking, dizziness, loss of balance, or coordination
- Sudden trouble seeing in one or both eyes
- Sudden unexplained severe headache

Prevention

There are several interventions that can prevent strokes. These include anti-coagulants, such as low-molecular-weight heparin and the anticoagulant warfarin, and taking cholesterol-lowering statins (such as Lipitor), which have been shown to decrease the risk of stroke in otherwise healthy individuals. Finally, there are several lifestyle modifications you can make:

- Stop smoking

---

187   revolutionhealth.com/conditions/brain-nerves/stroke/risk-factors/hor-mone-replacement-therapy.
188   strokeassociation.org/presenter.jhtml?identifier=1020.
189   mayoclinic.com/health/stroke/DS00150/DSECTION=symptoms.

- Drink alcohol in moderation, if at all
- Exercise regularly
- Take low-dose aspirin (ask your doctor for the proper dosage)
- Take vitamin D supplements (talk to your doctor about this)

Treatments

Procedure to follow if you or your loved one has suffered a stroke:

Get to a hospital right away: there is a three-hour window to prevent permanent brain damage. A clot busting drug called tissue plasminogen activator (tPA) has been approved for treating ischemic stroke, and although half of all stroke patients could benefit from this drug, only 3 to 4 percent receive it. This is because of two reasons: patients wait longer than the three-hour window to get to the hospital, and many hospitals won't give the drug without a diagnosis of ischemic stroke. The diagnosis can be made with an MRI machine to rule out intracranial hemorrhage (indicative of hemorrhagic stroke). If the patient has hemorrhagic stroke, doctors are not inclined to give tPA, because it could cause more bleeding into the brain. In the absence of an MRI machine, and with symptoms of stroke, your chances of recovery are better taking tPA than doing nothing at all. *The American Stroke Association recommends ambulances take stroke victims to stroke centers.*

Fewer than three percent of people suffering the most common kind of stroke (ischemic) get the best treatment for that type of stroke. Do your homework and identify a designated stroke center in your area *before* you have a stroke, and make sure you tell your friends and family that you want to be sent there if you have a stroke—this is a matter of life and death. For information about stroke centers, see footnotes.[190,191] In most areas, there are no uniform guidelines for 9-1-1 dispatch and emergency medical service to get patients to a hospital that can provide the treatment they need. Demand that your ambulance driver take you to a stroke center.

Rehabilitation

Rehabilitation is a critical part of recovery for many stroke survivors. The effects of stroke may mean that you must change, relearn, or redefine how you live. Stroke rehabilitation helps you return to independent living. Most gains in a person's ability to function in the first thirty days after a stroke are

---

190   jointcommission.org/CertificationPrograms/Disease-SpecificCare/ DSCOrgs.

191   stroke.org/site/DocServer/Stroke_Center_List.pdf?docID=1741.

due to spontaneous recovery. However, many researchers have seen progress years after suffering a stroke in the patients' ability to walk if they are given a form of physical therapy that uses a treadmill.[192]

Rehabilitation doesn't reverse the effects of a stroke. Its goals are to build your strength, capability, and confidence so you can continue your daily activities despite the effects of your stroke.

What you do in rehabilitation depends on what you need to become independent. You may work to improve your independence in many areas. These include the following:

- Self-care skills, such as feeding, grooming, bathing, and dressing
- Mobility skills, such as transferring, walking, or self-propelling a wheelchair
- Communication skills in speech and language
- Cognitive skills, such as memory or problem-solving
- Social skills for interacting with other people

Rehabilitation will begin when your doctor determines that you're medically stable and able to benefit from it. Most rehabilitation services require a doctor's order. Rehabilitation services are provided in many different places:

- Acute care and rehabilitation hospitals
- Long-term care facilities
- At home, through home health agencies
- Outpatient facilities

For information about stroke—including rehabilitation, nursing homes, assisted living, insurance questions, financial assistance, support groups, and other concerns—visit the National Stroke Association and Resource Directory.[193]

You may be involved in rehabilitation in some or all of these settings. It depends on what your needs are and what type of rehabilitation program will be best for you.

What Is a Rehabilitation Program?

Under your doctor's direction, rehabilitation specialists come together to provide a treatment program specifically suited to your needs. Physicians who

192   nytimes.com/2008/09/02/health/02regi.html?_r=1&ref=health.
193   stroke.org/site/PageServer?pagename=Resource_Directory_list.

specialize in rehabilitation are called physiatrists. The number of services you receive will depend on your needs. Services may include the following:

- Rehabilitation nursing
- Physical therapy
- Occupational therapy
- Speech-language pathology
- Audiology
- Recreational therapy
- Nutritional care
- Rehabilitation counseling
- Social work
- Psychiatry/psychology
- Chaplaincy
- Patient/family education
- Support groups

Vocational evaluation, driver's training, and programs to improve your physical and emotional stamina so you can go back to work also may be part of your rehabilitation program.

How Can I Learn More?

Talk to your doctor, nurse, or healthcare professional. You can also call 1-888-4-STROKE (478-7653) and ask for the Stroke Family Support Network. If you've had a stroke or have heart disease, members of your family also may be at higher risk. It's important for them to make changes now to lower their risk.

In conclusion, stroke is the third leading cause of death in this country, but there are many things you can do to reduce your risk. Also you can reduce the complications of stroke by getting to the right care. Identify a stroke center in your community so you know where to be taken in case you suffer one. Rehabilitation is usually necessary after having a stroke. [194]

---

194   americanstrokeassociation.org/presenter.jhtml?identifier=1200037.

Chapter 10

Take Control of Diabetes

Objectives:
- To understand the risk factors for diabetes
- To recognize the symptoms of diabetes
- To understand the complications associated with diabetes
- To learn to manage your diabetes
- To understand your treatment options for diabetes

Actual case: As reported by Gina Kolata in the NY Times, August 20, 2007, "Looking Past Blood Sugar to Survive with Diabetes"

Forty-four-year-old John Smith found out he had diabetes by accident, after a urine test during a physical exam. Both his urine and blood had very high amounts of sugar. After this, John became fixated on his blood sugar; counting carbohydrates in his diet, taking pills to control his blood sugar, and self-monitoring his blood sugar. He thought everything would be fine; his blood sugar was under control. However, he never looked beyond his diabetes. He didn't control his blood cholesterol or blood pressure, leaving him at risk for a heart attack, the number one killer of diabetics. Mr. Smith should not feel alone; many patients with diabetes are not getting all the treatment they need. One afternoon he had chest pain that expanded to his neck, along his shoulder, and down to his biceps. He was having a major heart attack. Luckily he was sent to a hospital with a heart center and recovered. Later he said he thought he had covered all the bases by controlling his diabetes. He thought its biggest complications were blindness, kidney disease, or amputation. He had no idea that heart disease was a major complication. He didn't know that he should treat his high cholesterol or blood pressure; in fact, his doctor never mentioned how important it was to control cholesterol levels or blood pressure. He left the hospital with a whole new drug regimen: a statin to drive down his cholesterol, two drugs to lower his blood pressure, an aspirin, insulin, and two drugs to reduce his blood sugar. This is what he should have been taking all along.

Common Myths about Diabetes

Myth: As long as I control my blood sugar I'll be fine.
Fact: Nearly all people with diabetes die from cardiovascular disease. It is not enough to just control your blood sugar; you must lower your cholesterol and bring down your blood pressure.

Myth: Taking insulin cures diabetes.
Fact: Insulin helps manage diabetes. It does not cure diabetes.

Myth: Fruit is a healthy food; therefore, I can eat as much as I want.
Fact: Yes, fruit is healthy, but it contains sugar and must be part of your diabetic meal plan.

Diabetes Definitions[195,196]

Diabetes is an incurable but treatable disease where the body does not produce or properly use insulin. Insulin is a hormone that is needed to convert sugar, starches, and other food into energy needed for daily life. The cause of diabetes continues to be a mystery, although both genetics and environmental factors such as obesity and lack of exercise play key roles.

Type 1 diabetes, previously known as juvenile diabetes, is usually diagnosed in children and young adults. In type 1 diabetes, the body does not produce insulin. Type 1 is lethal unless insulin is given via injections to replace the missing hormone.

Type 2 diabetes, or adult onset or non-insulin dependent diabetes, is the most common form of diabetes. In type 2 diabetes, either the body does not produce enough insulin or the cells ignore the insulin that is produced. It is often managed by engaging in exercise and modifying one's diet. It is rapidly increasing in the developed world, and there is some evidence that this pattern will be followed in much of the rest of the world in coming years.

Pre-diabetes is a condition that occurs when a person's blood glucose levels are higher than normal but not high enough for a diagnosis of type 2 diabetes. There are 57 million Americans who have pre-diabetes, in addition to the 23.6 million with diabetes. If you have pre-diabetes, the long-term damage of diabetes—especially to your heart and circulatory system—may already be starting. However, progression from pre-diabetes to type 2 diabetes isn't inevitable. With healthy lifestyle changes you may be able to bring your blood sugar level back to normal.

Gestational diabetes occurs immediately after pregnancy; 5 percent to 10 percent of women with gestational diabetes are found to have diabetes, usually type 2.[197]

---

195   diabetes.org.

196   mayoclinic.com/health/diabetes/DS01121.

197   diabeticdietsnews.com/gestational-diabetes-statistics/.

Risk Factors for Developing Type 1 (Juvenile) Diabetes[198]

Type 1 diabetes is most often diagnosed in children and young adults. The risk factors for developing type 1 diabetes are as follows:

- Family history: anyone with a sibling or parent with type 1 diabetes is at increased risk.
- Genetics: the presence of certain genes indicates a certain risk. Genetic testing of persons with a family history of type 1 diabetes can be done to determine the risk.
- Viral exposure may trigger an autoimmune response to pancreatic islet cells.

Risk Factors for Developing Type 2 Diabetes

Starting at puberty, if you're overweight or obese, have your blood sugar measured at least every three years. Normal fasting blood glucose levels generally run between 70 and 99 mg/dL. A value greater than 126 on two separate occasions generally means you have diabetes.

- A body mass index (BMI) below 18.5 is underweight; 18.5 to 24.9 is normal; 25 to 29.9 is considered overweight; and 30 and over is obese. Calculate you BMI with an online calculator.[199]
- The more fatty tissue you have the more chance you have to become insulin resistant.

If your body fat is unevenly distributed around your waist (so-called, apple-shape), regardless of your BMI, you're at increased risk for developing diabetes. Have your blood sugar measured every three years beginning at puberty. A waist-hip ratio greater than 0.9 for men and less than 0.8 for women increases your risk.

A family history of diabetes or a family background that is African American, American Indian, Asian American, Pacific Islander, or Hispanic American/Latino also raises your risk. If you've had gestational diabetes, or gave birth to at least one baby weighing more than 9 pounds, you're also at risk.

---

198   mayoclinic.com/health/type-1-diabetes-in-children/DS00931/ DSECTION=risk-factors.

199   bmi-calculator.net/.

> ## To calculate your risk, go to diabetes.org/ risk-test.jsp.

Metabolic syndrome is a cluster of conditions that occur together, increasing your risk of heart disease, stroke, and diabetes.[200] These conditions include:

- High blood pressure
- High blood cholesterol
- High blood sugar
- Insulin resistance
- Fat concentrated in the abdomen

If you have metabolic syndrome or any of the components of metabolic syndrome, you have the opportunity to make aggressive lifestyle changes. Making these changes can delay or derail the development of serious diseases that may result from metabolic syndrome.

Recognize the Risks Associated with Type 1 and Type 2 Diabetes

- Blindness
- Kidney disease
- Heart disease
- Stroke
- Hypertension
- Peripheral neuropathy
- Numbness or reduced ability to feel pain or changes in temperature, especially in your feet
- A tingling, burning or prickling sensation that starts in your toes or the balls of your feet and gradually spreads upward
- Sharp, jabbing or electric shock, such as pain that's worse at night
- Extreme sensitivity to the lightest touch—for some people, even the weight of a sheet can be agonizing
- Loss of balance and coordination
- Muscle weakness and difficulty walking
- Serious foot problems, such as ulcers, infections, deformities, and bone and joint pain

---

200   www.medicinenet.com/metabolic_syndrome/article.htm.

- Amputation, the result of poor circulation that often accompanies diabetes
- Dental disease

Symptoms of Diabetes

For a symptom checkup, visit the Mayo Clinic Web site.[201] See your doctor if you have,

- Frequent urination
- Excessive thirst
- Extreme hunger
- Unusual weight loss
- Increased fatigue
- Irritability
- Blurry vision
- Slow healing sores or infections
- Tingling hands and feet

Diabetes Complications

The longer you wait to be diagnosed with diabetes the greater your chance of already having some of its complications at time of diagnosis. These include:

- Cardiovascular disease
  - o Many patients have cardiovascular disease prior to being diagnosed with diabetes.
  - o Diabetics have a two to five times greater risk of developing cardiovascular disease.
  - o 70 percent of diabetic patients die from cardiovascular disease.[202]
  - o Lowering cholesterol levels reduces the risk of dying from heart attack by 30 to 40 percent.
  - o Many doctors believe that LDL cholesterol should be less than 80 mg/dL in patients with diabetes (normal less than

---

201   mayoclinic.com/health/symptom-checker/DS00671.
202   diabetes.webmd.com/news/20070611/diabetes-early-heart-disease-death?ecd=wnl_epi_061707.

100 mg/dL)

- On average, fifty-year-old men with diabetes have a shorter life expectancy of 21.3 years—7.5 years less than other men[1]
  - o These men develop heart disease in 14.2 years—7.8 years sooner than other men

- On average, fifty-year-old women with diabetes,
  - o Have a shorter life expectancy of 26.5 years—8.2 years less than that of other women
  - o These women develop heart disease in 19.6 years—8.4 years sooner than other women

Diagnosis

Diabetes is diagnosed on the basis of sustained high blood sugar. Patients are given a fasting plasma glucose test. You cannot eat or drink for at least eight hours before the test. A value of 126 mg/dL or greater must be verified by another test on another day before a diagnosis of diabetes can be made. This test is recommended for the diagnosis of diabetes.[203]

Table 10.1 Fasting blood glucose test

Plasma sugar (mg/dL)	Diagnosis
99 and below	Normal
100 to 125	Pre-diabetes (impaired fasting glucose)
126 and above	Diabetes

Source: diabetes.niddk.nih.gov/dm/pubs/diagnosis/#3

An *oral glucose tolerance test* measures your blood glucose after you have gone at least eight hours without eating and two hours after you drink a glucose-containing beverage. A value of 200 mg/dL or greater should must be verified by another test on another day before a diagnosis of diabetes can be made.

Table 10.2 Oral glucose tolerance test

---

203   professional.diabetes.org/Disease_Backgrounder.aspx?MID=233&RD=1.

2-Hour blood glucose result (mg/dL)	Diagnosis
139 and below	Normal
140 to 199	Pre-diabetes (impaired glucose tolerance)
200 and above	Diabetes

Source: diabetes.niddk.nih.gov/dm/pubs/diagnosis/#3

A randomized blood glucose test that reveals a blood glucose level of 200 mg/dL or more, or a glycosylated hemoglobin (hemoglobin A1C) greater than 7 percent are also forms of diagnoses. A1C measures the amount of sugar that has bound to hemoglobin, the substance that carries oxygen inside red blood cells in your blood. A1C is routinely used to help patients manage their diabetes.[204] The higher your average blood sugar level for the past two or three months, the higher your A1C levels.

Measuring control of blood glucose: In the presence of excess blood glucose, the hemoglobin ß-chain becomes increasingly glycosylated, making the A1C measurement a useful index of glycemic control. The importance of A1C as an index of diabetes control was reinforced by the Diabetes Control and Complications Trial (DCCT).[205] This study demonstrated a direct correlation between glycemic control as indicated by A1C and the likelihood of developing long-term diabetes-related complications.

Prevention [206,207,208]

Primary prevention: Type 1 diabetes cannot be prevented; however, the same healthy lifestyle choices that have been discussed throughout this book can help prevent prediabetes, type 2 diabetes, and gestational diabetes. [3]

Lifestyle changes have been shown to reduce the risk of developing diabetes by 58 percent![209] The goal of lifestyle intervention is to achieve and maintain 7 percent or greater weight loss through a low-calorie, low-fat diet and 150 or more minutes of moderate physical activity weekly. Criteria for lifestyle changes:

204   diabetesforums.com/forum/lo-fi/t-35954.html.

205   bsc.gwu.edu/bsc/studies/dcct.html.

206   mayoclinic.com/health/diabetes/DS01121/DSECTION=prevention.

207   "Summary of revisions for the 2009 Clinical Practice Recommendations. *Diabetes Care* 32: 53, 2009.

208   healthierus.gov/steps/summit/prevportfolio/strategies/reducing/diabetes/prevention.htm.

209   "Primary Prevention of Type 2 Diabetes Mellitus by Lifestyle Changes: Implications for Health Policy" *Annals of Internal Medicine* 140: 951, 2004.

- Overweight (BMI greater than 85th percentile for age and sex, weight for height greater than 85th percentile or weigh greater than 120 percent of ideal for height). *Plus any of two of the following risk factors:*
  - o Family history of type 2 diabetes in first or second-degree relative
  - o Race/ethnicity (Native American, African American, Latino, Asian American, Pacific Islander)
  - o Signs of insulin resistance or conditions associated with insulin resistance (hypertension, high cholesterol or triglycerides)
- For a BMI calculator, see, bmi-calculator.net
- For a calorie counter see, nytimes.com/ref/health/caloriecounter. html
- Ask your doctor about the Glycemic Index Diet to help manage your diabetes.

If lifestyle changes do not work, patients should talk to their doctor about oral hypoglycemic therapy. If oral hypoglycemic therapy is not successful, the patient should talk to their doctor about insulin. Fasting blood sugar levels should be under 100 mg/dL. Patients should strive for hemoglobin A1C levels less than 7 percent.

Note: There is a sub-group of diabetic patients over 55 years of age with cardiovascular disease or risk factors for cardiovascular disease that should have more moderate blood glucose control with hemoglobin A1C levels of 7 to 8 percent.[210] A semi-annual glucose A1C test will ensure your diabetes is being managed properly.

Secondary and tertiary prevention focuses on people with diabetes and seeks to prevent (secondary) or control (tertiary) the devastating complications of this disease. More proven intervention models are available for both secondary and tertiary prevention than for primary prevention. [211]

You should have an examination twice a year by your primary care doctor in which your blood pressure is taken, blood is drawn for a lipid panel, and sugar levels are measured. If you are changing medications or cannot control your blood sugar it is recommended that the blood glucose test be done four times a year. If your blood pressure and/or cholesterol are high you must be

---

210   diabetes.org/for-media/pr-ada-statement-related-to-accord-trail-announce-ment-020608.jsp.

211   mayoclinic.com/health/diabetes/DS01121/DSECTION=prevention

given medications to lower them. Your LDL cholesterol should be under 100 mg/dL and your blood pressure should be less than 130/80 mm Hg.

If protein is found in your urine, talk to your doctor about taking an angiotensin converting enzyme (ACE) inhibitor. Also, have an annual eye by an opthamologist or optometrist to look for damage to blood vessels from the diabetes which could result in blindness (diabetic retinopathy). Have your feet examined twice a year to look for evidence of diabetic neuropathy, and have a dental exam twice a year because diabetics are at risk for periodontal disease.

Other ways to prevent the complications of diabetes include:

- Quit smoking.
- Identify sores that won't go away—call your doctor.
- Learn ways to manage stress.
- If you are on insulin therapy, measure your blood sugar with a home monitoring device as instructed by your doctor.
- Take all your medications and refill your medications. You will be taking these medications for the rest of your life.
- If you experience any side effects from your medications, talk to your doctor. *Do not stop taking any medications without first speaking with your doctor.*
- If you are over forty, talk with your doctor about taking a baby aspirin (81 mg) daily.
- Work with your healthcare professional, which may include nutritionists, personal trainers, as well as doctors and nurses to ensure a long and healthy life.

Recently, the Centers for Disease Control and Prevention reported that the number of Americans with diabetes had grown to about 24 million, with people sixty and over accounting for 25 percent of the cases. There are 23.6 million children and adults in the United States, or 7.8 percent of the population, who have diabetes. While an estimated 17.9 million have been diagnosed with diabetes, 5.7 million people (or nearly one quarter) are unaware that they have the disease, because they do not recognize the symptoms. But you don't need to become a statistic. Understanding symptoms listed above can lead to early diagnosis and treatment—and a lifetime of better health.

In the United States, an additional 54 million adults have pre-diabetes, according to the American Diabetes Association. Without intervention, pre-diabetes is likely to become type 2 diabetes in as little as ten years. Pre-diabetes is a condition in which your blood sugar level is higher than normal, but not high enough to be classified as type 2 diabetes. Still, the stakes are high. If you have pre-diabetes, the long-term damage of diabetes—especially to your heart and circulatory system—may already be starting. Progression from pre-diabetes to type 2 diabetes isn't inevitable. With healthy lifestyle changes—such as eating healthy foods, including physical activity in your daily routine, and maintaining a healthy weight—you may be able to bring your blood sugar level back to normal.

Obesity does increase the risk of developing diabetes, but the disease involves more than being obese. Only 5 percent to 10 percent of obese people have diabetes, and many who have diabetes are not obese. To a large extent, type 2 diabetes is genetically determined—if one identical twin has it, the other has an 80 percent chance of having it too.

- Many of the long term complications of diabetes such as neuropathy, blindness, and kidney disease can be prevented or delayed with intensive glucose control (A1C less than 7.0). These complications include:
- Blindness
- Kidney failure
- Amputations (neuropathy)
- Frailty and fractures

Children and Diabetes

As many as 30 percent of children and adolescents are overweight and are at increased risk for diabetes.[212] There are new guidelines for childhood obesity. Weight awareness offers the best hope for preventing overweight- and obesity-associated disease progression with its associated morbidities into adulthood.

At checkup, overweight and obese children (with BMIs in the 85th to 95th percentile and greater than 95th percentile, respectively) must be given specific diet and exercise guidelines and short follow-up times. Educating families about energy-dense foods and sweetened beverages will help, as will recommending at least sixty minutes of moderate physical activity a day for all family members.

Thousands of children are taking adult medications for chronic conditions related to obesity. These include

- Drugs to treat high blood pressure
- Drugs to treat high cholesterol
- Drugs to treat type 2 diabetes

People who develop type 2 diabetes before the age twenty are more likely to develop end-stage kidney disease and die in middle age, compared to people who develop the disease at a later age, a study has revealed.[213]

---

212   weightawareness.com/common/print.xml?document_id=1176.
213   diabetes.niddk.nih.gov/dm/pubs/statistics/.

Chapter 11

Take Control of Cancer

Objectives
- To understand what cancer is
- To understand what causes cancer
- To understand the risk factors that may increase your chance of cancer
- To understand the screening, diagnosis, and treatment of cancer
- To know the right questions to ask so you get the right care
- To understand how cancer may be prevented

Actual case: As reported by Denise Grady in the *NY Times*, July 29, 2007, "Cancer Patients Lost in a Maze of Uneven Care"

The first doctor gave her six months to live. The second and third said chemotherapy would buy more time, but surgery would not. A fourth offered to operate. Karen had just given birth to her first child last July when doctors discovered she had colon cancer. She was only thirty-five, and the disease had already spread to her liver. The months she had hoped to spend getting to know her new daughter were hijacked by illness, fear, and a desperate quest to survive. For the past year she traveled from coast to coast trying to find the care that would allow her to watch her daughter take her first steps.

"It's patchwork, and frustrating that there's not one person taking care of me who I can look to as my champion," Karen said recently in a telephone interview from her home near Seattle. "I don't feel I have a doctor who is looking out for my care. My oncologist is terrific, but he's an oncologist. The surgeon seems terrific, but I found him through my own diligence. I have no confidence in the system."

"I think I'd be dead if I'd stayed with the first provider," she said. She rejected the first oncologist and, with persistence and good health insurance, Karen found the right care, and was there when her baby took her first steps.

Myth: Cancer is almost always fatal.
Fact: Because of new treatment breakthroughs and earlier detection before the cancer is untreatable, nearly 40 percent of cancer patients reach or exceed the five-year survival rate.

Cancer Definitions[214]

- **Oncology** is the branch of medicine that studies cancer.
- **Cancer** is the common term for all malignant tumors. It is characterized as the uncontrolled, abnormal growth of cells.
- **Risk factors** are anything that increases someone's chance of getting a disease.
- **Genetics** is the study of how traits and diseases are passed from one generation to the next.

---

214   cancer.net/patient/Learning+About+Cancer.

- **Tumor staging** is the process of describing the size and location of the tumor(s) and determining whether the cancer has spread to other parts of the body.
- **Radiation therapy** is the use of high-energy X-rays or other particles to kill cancer cells. If you need radiation therapy, you will be asked to see a specialist called a radiation oncologist.
- **Chemotherapy** is the use of drugs to kill cancer cells. It is given by an internist who is a specialist in cancer, called an *oncologist*. The side effects of chemotherapy depend on the individual and the drug and the dose used, but can include fatigue, hair loss, risk of infection, nausea and vomiting, loss of appetite, and diarrhea. These side effects usually go away once treatment is finished.
- **Adjuvant therapy** is treatment that is given after surgery to lower the risk of the cancer returning. Adjuvant therapy includes radiation therapy, chemotherapy, and targeted therapy.
- **Targeted therapy** is a treatment that targets faulty genes or proteins that contribute to cancer growth and development. These drugs are becoming more important in the treatment of certain cancers, such as breast cancer and colorectal cancer.

The most common cancers facing Americans will be discussed in detail following some general information that pertains to all cancers.

Overall Risk Factors for Cancer

There is much still to be learned about cancer. Hopefully, with the sequencing of the human genome completed, we will make great progress in our understanding of the disease over the next decade.

Most cancers come from mutations to genes, viruses, or tobacco use. Cancer is a disease of aging, since most cancers occur in people over sixty-five.

It is uncommon for cancers to run in families; however, there are a few that seem to run more in families than the rest of the population. For example,

- Melanoma, breast, prostate, colorectal, and ovarian cancer
- Inherited gene changes, mutations of genes
- BRCA1 and BRCA 2 genes for breast cancer
- Familial Adenomatous Polyposis (FAP) for colorectal cancer

Tobacco products such as chewing tobacco and snuff lead to cancer of the head and neck. Smoking tobacco or being around tobacco smoke (passive and environmental) can cause cancer of the lung, larynx, mouth, throat, esophagus, bladder, kidney, stomach, pancreas, colon, and cervix.

Ultraviolet irradiation from sunlight, sunlamps, and tanning booths increases the risk of early aging of the skin, skin damage, and cancers of the skin, such as basal cell carcinoma, squamous cell carcinoma, and the deadliest form of skin cancer, melanoma.

Consuming more than two alcoholic drinks per day for many years increases the risk of cancer of the mouth, throat, esophagus, larynx, liver, colon, rectum, and breast. The risk is even higher if you smoke on top of drinking alcohol.

Poor diet, lack of physical activity, being overweight or obese, and socioeconomic status (a composite construct of income, wealth, education, employment, and residential neighborhood) increase the risk of colorectal cancer and breast cancer. Being poor increases the risk of being diagnosed at a later (more aggressive and harder to treat) stage of the cancer.

Some *viruses* and *bacteria*, such as the Human papilloma viruses (HPV), are known to cause cancer of the cervix, throat, and anus. Hepatitis B and hepatitis C cause cancer of the liver. Other viruses and bacteria that can cause cancer include,

- Human immunodeficiency virus (HIV) (lymphoma, Kaposi's sarcoma)
- Epstein Barr Virus (EBV) (lymphoma)
- *Helicobacter pylori* (cancers of the stomach)

Smoking and smokeless tobacco are the major culprits in a multitude of cancers beyond lung cancer, such cancer of the oral cavity, pharynx, larynx, esophagus, bladder, stomach, cervix, kidney and pancreas, and acute myeloid leukemia.

Risk Reduction/Prevention of Cancer

Many cancers are preventable. For example, tobacco use is the leading cause of death from cancer in the United States, with 175,000 cancer deaths each year.[215]

Heavy alcohol usage has been associated with cancer of the esophagus, pharynx, and mouth, whereas a more controversial association links alcohol

---

215   quitsmoking.about.com/od/tobaccostatistics/a/cancerstats.htm.

with liver, breast, and colorectal cancer.[216] The Dietary Guidelines for Americans 2005 emphasize moderation for those who choose to drink, moderation "defined as the consumption of up to one drink a day for women and up to two drinks a day for men."[217]

Obesity is a risk factor for cancers of the colon, breast, endometrium (lining of the uterus), kidney, prostate, and esophagus.[218] This can be avoided by leading a healthier lifestyle with better nutrition and more exercise. Too much red meat and processed foods have been associated with certain cancers. Eat a diet rich in fiber and whole grains and low in fat.

Cancer Diagnosis

If you are diagnosed with cancer, be sure your primary care doctor refers you to a board-certified oncologist, surgical oncologist, or radiation oncologist who is affiliated with a cancer center.[219,220]

If you are diagnosed with cancer, always get a *second opinion* from an expert. Approximately 30 percent of second opinions disagree with the first diagnosis. An expert is someone who routinely treats your particular tumor type.

Doctors use many tests to diagnose cancer and determine if the cancer has metastasized (spread). Some tests may also determine which treatments may be the most effective. For most types of cancer, examination of a biopsy by a pathologist is the only way to make a definitive diagnosis of cancer. Be sure to get a second opinion from a pathologist who examines cancers such as yours on a routine basis (i.e., hundreds of times). If a biopsy is not possible, the doctor may suggest other tests that will help make a diagnosis. Imaging tests may be used to find out whether the cancer has metastasized. Your doctor may consider these factors when choosing a diagnostic test:

- Your age and medical condition
- The type of cancer suspected
- Severity of symptoms
- Previous test results

---

216   alcoholism.about.com/cs/alerts/l/blnaa21.htm.

217   drinkingandyou.com/site/us/moder.htm.

218   obesityfocused.com/articles/obesity-and-cancer/index.php.

219   Abms.org.

220   nci.nih.gov.

Cancer Prevention

One third of all cancers are due to controllable, modifiable factors![221] Cancer prevention is taking action to lower the chance of getting cancer. To prevent new cancers from starting, scientists look at risk factors and protective factors. Anything that increases your chance of developing cancer is called a cancer "risk factor"; anything that decreases your chance of developing cancer is called a cancer "protective factor."

Some risk factors for cancer can be avoided, but many cannot. For example, both smoking and inheriting certain genes are risk factors for some types of cancer, but only smoking can be avoided. Avoiding risk factors and increasing protective factors may lower your risk, but it does not mean that you will not get cancer.

Despite scientific evidence that cancer deaths can be reduced by modifying risky behavior and by cancer screening, a significant portion of the population ignores having these tests:

- Approximately 16 percent of women have not had a Pap test in the previous three years.[222]
- Approximately 50 percent of people over fifty have not had a colonoscopy or sigmoidoscopy.[223]
- Approximately 76 percent of people over fifty have not had a blood stool test in previous two years.[224]
- One in three women over forty have not had a mammogram in previous two years.[225]
- 20 percent of people still smoke cigarettes[226]
- 15.4 percent of people reported binge drinking[227]
- 26 percent of people over twenty are obese due to poor diet and lack of exercise.[228]

Recommended Cancer Screening

The U.S. Preventive Services Task Force[229] (referred to here as the "Task Force") is an independent panel of experts in the fields of family medicine,

221   healthyone.org/?cat=187.
222   meps.ahrq.gov/mepsweb/data_files/publications/st173/stat173.pdf.
223   Fightcolore ctalcancer.org/tag/screening/page/4.
224   doh.sd.gov/Statistics/2006BRFSS/Colorectal.pdf.
225   rsna.org/media/pressreleases/pr_target.cfm?ID=195.
226   cnn.com/2009/HEALTH/01/09/who.still.smokes/.
227   pubs.niaaa.nih.gov/publications/AA67/AA67.htm.
228   obesity1.tempdomainname.com/subs/fastfacts/obesity_US.shtml.
229   preventiveservices.ahrq.gov.

obstetrics-gynecology, cancer, pediatrics, nursing, prevention research, and psychology that evaluates randomized, controlled clinical trials for the benefits of cancer screening. The Task Force recommends screening for the following cancers, since screening asymptomatic people decreases the death rate from these cancers:

- Cervical cancer
- Breast cancer
- Skin cancer
- Colorectal cancer (cancer of the colon and rectum)
- Prostate cancer (only after thoughtful discussion with your doctor)

Each of these cancers will be discussed in detail below. THE TASK FORCE *DOES NOT RECOMMEND* ROUTINE SCREENING FOR THE FOLLOWING CANCERS BECAUSE SCREENING HAD NO EFFECT ON SURVIVAL:

o Bladder cancer
o Ovarian cancer
o Genetic screening for ovarian cancer (unless you have increased risk for deleterious mutations of the breast cancer susceptibility gene BRAC1 or BRAC2, genetic counseling is recommended)
o Lung cancer—there is not conclusive evidence that screening for lung cancer prevents deaths or not, therefore, the task force cannot recommend for or against routine screening using either low dose computerized tomography, chest X-ray, or sputum cytology
o Oral cancer—evidence insufficient to recommend for or against screening
o Pancreatic cancer

Treatment Options for Cancer

One problem with cancer treatment is that the care is often uneven and complicated, leaving the patient out of the decision-making process. It is important to have a primary care physician who can coordinate your treatments among the various oncology specialties.

There are many treatment options, depending on the stage and grade of your particular cancer. The latest treatment options for 70 percent to 80 percent of cancers can be found at the National Cancer Comprehensive

Network.[230] Go to their Web site and enter the type of cancer you want information about in the search box.

Most people don't often think to ask the pathologist examining their biopsy (or the radiologist examining their mammogram) whether they have a lot of experience with diagnosing a particular type of cancer. To be an expert, the pathologist should have examined so many cases (literally hundreds) that is has become routine in their practice. Go to an institution where diagnosis and treatment of your particular tumor is routine and ask the right questions to get the right treatment. Some of these questions are listed below:

- How often do you read these types of X-rays?
- How often have you treated this type of cancer? Once? Two hundred times? You want someone who has done it hundreds of times.
- How often do you perform this type of surgery?
- How many of these procedures have you performed?
- What's the overall success rate for this type of surgery?
- What's the success rate for those surgeries that you've performed?

Talk to your doctor about treatment options that work well for you.

Cervical Cancer[231]

The American Cancer Society estimates that in 2009, about 11,270 cases of invasive cervical cancer will be diagnosed in the United States, which will result in about 4,000 deaths.[232] Cervical cancer was once one of the most common causes of cancer death for American women. The cervical cancer death rate declined by 74 percent between 1955 and 1992 thanks to the increased use of the Pap test. This screening procedure can find changes in the cervix before cancer develops. It can also find early cervical cancer in its most curable stage. The death rate from cervical cancer continues to decline by nearly 4 percent a year.

Cervical cancer tends to occur in midlife. Most cases are found in women younger than fifty. It rarely develops in women younger than twenty. Many older women do not realize that the risk of developing cervical cancer is still present as they age. Almost 20 percent of women with cervical cancer are

---

230   nccn.org.

231   cancer.net/patient/Cancer+Types/Cervical+Cancer.

232   cancer.org/docroot/CRI/content/CRI_2_4_1X_What_are_the_key_statis-
       tics_for_cervical_cancer_8.asp?rnav=cri.

diagnosed when they are over sixty-five. That is why it is important for older women to continue having regular Pap tests.

Prevention and Risk Reduction

- HPV vaccination. The American Cancer Society[233] recommends vaccinating women eleven to eighteen years of age.
- Limiting the number of sexual partners.
- Avoiding sexual intercourse with people who have had many partners.
- Avoiding sexual intercourse with people who are obviously infected with genital warts or show other symptoms.
- Having safe sex by using condoms will reduce the risk of HPV infection. Condoms also protect against HIV and AIDS.
- Avoiding smoking.

Symptoms of Cervical Cancer

Most women do not display symptoms until the cancer has spread to other tissues. Any of the following could be signs or symptoms of precancerous changes or cancer; if you recognize them, see your doctor immediately:

- Blood spots or light bleeding between or following periods
- Menstrual bleeding that is longer and heavier than usual
- Bleeding after intercourse, douching, or a pelvic examination
- Pain during sexual intercourse
- Bleeding after menopause
- Increased vaginal discharge

Cervical Cancer Screening

Cervical screening using the Pap test has reduced the mortality rates from cervical cancer by 75 percent since its implementation in 1949.[234]
- Pap test and HPV test for cervical cancer screening[235]
- Beginning at age thirty, women who have had three normal Pap test results in a row may get screened every two to three years.

---

233   guidelines.gov/summary/summary.aspx?doc_id=11876.
234   cancer.org/docroot/CRI/content/CRI_2_4_4X_Surgery_8.asp?rnav=cri.
235   cancer.org/docroot/CRI/content/CRI_2_4_3X_Can_cervical_cancer_be_ found_early_8.asp?rnav=cri.

- Women seventy years of age or older who have had three or more normal Pap tests in a row and no abnormal Pap test results in the last ten years may choose to stop having cervical cancer screening.
- Women with a history of cervical cancer, DES exposure before birth, HIV infection, or a weakened immune system should continue to have screening as long as they are in good health.
- Women who have had a total hysterectomy (removal of the uterus and cervix) may also choose to stop having cervical cancer screening, unless the surgery was done as a treatment for cervical cancer or pre-cancer. Women who have had a hysterectomy without removal of the cervix should continue to follow the guidelines above.
- To find an expert pathologist, call a medical school near you and ask for an expert in the Department of Pathology, or call a cancer center in your area for a second opinion.[236]
- For state of the art treatment, go to a designated cancer center near you.[1]

> **If you are diagnosed with cervical cancer get a second opinion from a pathologist for whom examining cervical cancer is routine.**

Diagnostic Tests[237]

A pelvic exam is a digital exam to feel if there are any abnormalities in the cervix and uterus, and to examine the ovaries. A colposcopy uses an instrument to examine the vagina and cervix. A colposcopy isn't used unless the pelvic exam is abnormal. If a biopsy is called for, a small amount a tissue will be removed. Virtually 70 percent of cervical cancers are caused by infection with HPV 16 or HPV 18.[238] HPV can be used in women over thirty along with the Pap smear as a screening test. In women under thirty, HPV is used to triage abnormal Pap smears.

Treatment

Electrosurgical excision procedure (LEEP) is an office procedure used to remove precancerous lesions. A *cone biopsy* is done in the hospital to remove precancerous lesions. If more invasive cancer is seen, you and your doctor

---

236   nci.nih.gov.
237   cancer.org/docroot/CRI/content/CRI_2_4_4X_Surgery_8.asp?rnav=cri.
238   cancer.org/docroot/CRI/content/CRI_2_4_2X_What_are_the_risk_fac-tors_for_cervical_cancer_8.asp?rnav=cri.

will have to decide on how to proceed. Talk to your doctor about a treatment that works well for you.

Chemotherapy and radiation therapy is also used in some circumstances. For the right treatment, see a board-certified gynecologic oncologist. Visit abms.org to find one in your area.

> **It is very important for you to discuss your treatment options with your doctor.**

Breast Cancer[239]

The American Cancer Society estimates 192,000 new cases of invasive breast cancer and 40,000 deaths in the United States for 2009.[240]

Other than skin cancer, breast cancer is the most common cancer among women in the United States. It is the second leading cause of cancer death in women, after lung cancer.

The chance of a woman having invasive breast cancer some time during her life is about 1 in 8. The chance of dying from breast cancer is about 1 in 35. Breast cancer death rates are going down. This is probably the result of early detection and improved treatment. Right now, there are about two and a half million breast cancer survivors in the United States.

Prevention and Reduction of Risks

There are several risk factors for breast cancer:

- *Age.* Breast cancer shows an exponential rise until menopause followed by a slower increase.[241]
- *Obesity*
- *Family history.* Breast cancer in mother, sister, or daughter.
- *Breast density.* Tissue-to-fat ratio among women forty and older. Denser breasts may mean greater breast cancer risk.[242] Breast density is determined by mammography.
- *History of atypical hyperplasia (precancerous changes) on a breast biopsy.*

---

239   cancer.net/patient/Cancer+Types/Breast+Cancer.
240   cancer.org/docroot/CRI/content/CRI_2_2_1X_How_many_people_get_
breast_cancer_5.asp?sitearea=.
241   cancersupportivecare.com/breastage1.html#abstract.
242   webmd.com/cancer/brain-cancer/news/20070117/breast-density-cancer-
link.

- *Hormone replacement therapy (HRT).* Used to reduce the symptoms of menopause, this combination of the female hormones progestin and estrogen is associated with an increased risk of breast cancer. HRT should only be used as a last resort and only after consultation with your doctor. It should only be taken for the shortest time possible at the lowest dose.

The risk for developing breast cancer within the next five years can be estimated, using risk factor information, by completing the National Cancer Institute Breast Cancer Risk Tool (the "Gail model," or by calling 800-4-CANCER).[243]

Women with a personal or family history of breast tumors must work with their physicians and schedule more frequent exams. However, breast tissue in younger women (younger than thirty years) tends to be denser, and this makes it more difficult to detect small changes in the breast on a mammogram. These women may be screened for breast tumors by means of echography or ultrasound once every two to three years. As women get older, the breast becomes less dense and X-rays are clearer.

Women with a family history of breast or ovarian cancer that includes a relative with a mutation in the BRCA1/BRCA2 breast cancer susceptibility genes should be referred for genetic counseling. Prophylactic mastectomy has been shown to reduce the risk of breast cancer by 95 percent in women with the BRCA mutation.

Women who are at higher than normal risk for developing breast cancer may consider chemoprevention (the use of drugs to reduce breast cancer risk). One such drug is tamoxifen (Nolvadex), a selective estrogen receptor modulator (SERM). A SERM is a medication that blocks estrogen receptors in some tissues and not others. Tamoxifen can reduce a woman's risk of developing breast cancer and the risk of the cancer recurring once a woman has been treated for breast cancer. Like estrogen, tamoxifen helps increase bone density in postmenopausal women and protects the cardiovascular system. Unlike estrogen, SERMs do not promote the development of breast cells into cancer cells; however, they may increase the risk of blood clots and uterine (endometrial) cancer.

Symptoms of Breast Cancer

Most women do not develop symptoms, so it is important to be aware of any changes to the breast. Some of these may include,

---

243   cancer.gov/bcrisktool/.

- New lumps (many women normally have lumpy breasts) or a thickening in the breast or under the arm
- Nipple tenderness, discharge, or physical changes (such as a nipple turned inward or a persistent sore)
- Skin irritation or changes, such as puckers, dimples, scaliness, or new creases
- Warm, red, swollen breasts with a rash resembling the skin of an orange
- Pain in the breast (usually not a symptom of breast cancer, but should be reported to a doctor)

Breast Cancer Screening[244]

The Task Force does not recommend teaching or performing self-examination, because it has not shown to increase survival.[245] The American Cancer Society considers self-examination an option to be determined by the patient and her doctor.

The Task Force does recommend a baseline mammogram in women thirty-five to forty years of age and a mammogram every three years until forty years of age. After forty, a mammogram should be done every one to two years. Get your mammogram done right—be sure your radiologist reads mammograms on a routine basis!

Radiologists misinterpreting mammograms is one of the leading causes malpractice litigation. Ask you OB/GYN to recommend a radiologist.

If you are diagnosed with breast cancer, get a *second opinion* from a pathologist who routinely examines breast cancer. One can be found at most medical schools or designated cancer centers.[246]

Diagnostic Tests

Your oncologist will determine your course of treatment after considering the following:

---

244   qap.sdsu.edu/screening/breastcancer/facts.html.
245   U.S. Preventive Services Task Force, "Screening for Breast Cancer: Recommendations and Rationale," *Annals of Internal Medicine*, 137 (5, part 1): 344–346.
246   nci.nih.gov.

- The stage and grade of the tumor
- The tumor's hormone receptor status (estrogen receptor, ER, progesterone receptor, PR), and HER2 status
- Your age and general health
- Your menopausal status
- The presence of known mutations to breast cancer genes

The Web site Adjuvant Online (adjuvantonline.com) is one such tool that your doctor can access to interpret a variety of prognostic factors. *This Web site should only be used with the assistance of your doctor.*

Treatment[247]

It is very important for you to discuss your treatment options with your doctor. The most common are surgery, radiation treatments, hormone therapy, and targeted therapy.

Surgery
The types of surgery are:

- Lumpectomy: removal of the tumor and a small area around the tumor that is clear of tumor.
- Total mastectomy: removing the entire breast, but not the underarm lymph nodes (sometimes called simple mastectomy). Women may also consider reconstruction surgery after this.
- Modified mastectomy: removal of breast and underarm lymph nodes.
- Axillary (underarm) lymph node dissection: removing the lymph nodes draining the breast and a pathologist examining them for tumor.
- Sentinel node biopsy: removing the first two or three lymph nodes that receives drainage from the breast.[248] If the sentinel nodes are free of cancer, it has been shown that the subsequent lymph nodes will be free of tumor and no further surgery is needed.

---

247   cancer.org/docroot/CRI/content/CRI_2_4_4X_How_Is_Breast_Cancer_ Treated_5.asp?rnav=cri.
248   cancer.net/patient/ASCO+Resources/What+to+Know   percent3A+ASCO percent27s+Guidelines/What+to+Know percent3A+ASCO percent27s+Guideli ne+on+Sentinel+Lymph+Node+Biopsy+in+Early+Stage+Breast+Cancer.

Radiation therapy

Radiation therapy is standard after *a lumpectomy* or *partial lumpectomy*. There has been growing interest in newer radiation methods to shorten the length of treatment from six to seven weeks to periods of three to four weeks. In one method (called hypo-fractionated radiation therapy), a higher daily dose is given to the whole breast each day so that the overall length of treatment is shortened to three to four weeks.

To lower risk of breast cancer recurrence, the doctor may use a combination of surgery with radiation:

- Lumpectomy or partial mastectomy and radiation therapy
- Total mastectomy, with or without immediate reconstruction, with or without sentinel node biopsy and possible axillary lymph node dissection
- Modified radical mastectomy with or without immediate reconstruction

Hormone Therapy

Estrogen stimulates the growth of about two out of three breast cancers that are PR or ER positive. Therefore, hormones that either block the effect of estrogen or lower estrogen levels are used to treat ER and PR positive breast cancers. Hormone therapy may be used as an adjuvant after radiation therapy.

Tamoxifen works by temporarily binding to and blocking estrogen from binding breast cancer cells. About 50 percent of the women taking tamoxifen for five years after surgery did not have recurrence of the tumor.

Aramatase inhibitors stop the small amount of estrogen production in post-menopausal women.

Targeted Therapy

Herceptin is approved for both the treatment of advanced breast cancer and as an adjuvant therapy for early-stage breast cancers that are HER2 positive. HER2 is a growth promoting protein.

Avastin is used to treat metastatic or recurrent breast cancer. This drug blocks the formation of new blood vessels which are necessary for tumor growth and metastasis.

Colorectal Cancer[249]

The American Cancer Society estimates 106,000 and 41,000 new cases of colon and rectal cancers, respectively, in the United States are for 2009. These will result in 49,000 deaths from colorectal cancer.[250]

Not counting skin cancers, colorectal cancer is the third most common cancer found in men and women in this country. The risk of a person having colorectal cancer in their lifetime is about 1 in 19. The death rate from colorectal cancer has been going down for the past fifteen years. One reason is there are fewer cases thanks to colorectal screening. Precancerous polyps can be found and removed before they turn into cancer. And colorectal cancer can also be found earlier when it is easier to cure. Treatments have improved as well.

Risk Factors and Prevention for Developing Colorectal Cancer

Many people with colorectal cancer experience no symptoms in the early stages of the disease. When symptoms appear, they may include a change in bowel habits, diarrhea, constipation, and bright red or very dark blood in the stool. Stools may appear narrower or thinner than normal, or you may experience bloating, gas pains, fullness, or cramps. You may feel constantly tired, experience unexplained weight loss, and unexplained iron deficiency anemia.[251]

Risk Factors
- Presence of adenomatous polyps by colonoscopy
- Age
- Inflammatory bowel disease
- Family history of colorectal cancer
- Smoking
- Obesity
- Race (colorectal cancer is the leading cause of cancer deaths in African Americans)
- Physical inactivity and obesity

---

249   cancer.net/patient/Cancer+Types/Colorectal+Cancer

250   [2]   cancer.org/docroot/CRI/content/CRI_2_2_1X_How_Many_People_Get_Colorectal_Cancer.asp?sitearea=.

251   mayoclinic.com/health/colon-cancer/DS00035/DSECTION=symptoms.

Prevention

- Non-steroidal anti-inflammatory drugs may reduce the development of polyps.
- Diets rich in fruits and vegetables and low in red meats may reduce the risk of colorectal cancer.

Screening for Colorectal Cancer[252,253]

Beginning at age fifty, the *preferred* screening test is colonoscopy, and it should be repeated every ten years, ending at age seventy-five. People eighty-five and over should not be screened. Between seventy-five and eighty-five, it's up to the patient and doctor whether to be screened. African Americans should be tested beginning at age of forty-five.

If you do not want to undergo a colonoscopy, you should consider an alternative cancer detection test, such as an annual hemaccult sensor, fecal DNA testing (every three years), a flexible sigmoidoscopy (every five to ten years), or a CT colonography (every five years). If polyps are found, they should be removed and examined for a malignancy. Discuss these screening options with your doctor.

> **Get the right care by going to a colorectal surgeon! To find one near you, go to abms.org.**

Diagnosis of Colorectal Cancer[254]

There are three types of diagnostic tools to detect colorectal cancer: biopsy, blood tests, and imaging.

With blood tests, the doctor is looking for

- Hemoglobin levels to determine whether you are anemic, which could be a result of bleeding into the colon
- Carcinoembryonic antigen (CEA), which might indicate that the cancer has spread to other parts of the body

---

252   ahrq.gov/clinic/uspstf/uspscolo.htm.
253   American College of Gastroenterology Guidelines for Colorectal Cancer Screening 2008 Am J Gastroenterol 104: 739, 2009.
254   cancer.net/patient/Cancer+Types/Colorectal+Cancer.

Imaging tests are used to determine whether the cancer has spread (metastasized) to other parts of the body.

If you are diagnosed with colorectal cancer, have your biopsy sent for a *second opinion* to a pathologist who routinely examines colorectal tumors. For the name of an expert, consult with the Department of Pathology at a local medical school in your area or call a cancer center in your area. Also, you can go to a designated cancer center for diagnosis and treatment. These centers have the expertise to make sure you get the right treatment.[255]

Be involved with your treatment so you get the right care.

Treatment

The treatment of colorectal cancer depends on the size and location of the tumor, whether the cancer has spread, and the patient's overall health. In many cases, a team of specialists, including a gastroenterologist (a doctor who specializes in the function and disorders of the gastrointestinal tract), surgeon, medical oncologist, and radiation oncologist will work with the patient to determine the best treatment plan, which may include the following:

- *Surgery*
    - o   Resection /anastomosis
    - o   Surgery to remove parts of other organs, such as the liver, lungs, and ovaries, where the cancer may have recurred or spread metastasized
- *Radiation therapy* or *chemotherapy* may be offered to some patients as palliative therapy to relieve symptoms and improve quality of life.
- *Clinical trials* of new chemotherapy and/or biologic therapy. For more specific results, refine the search by using other search features, such as the location of the trial, the type of treatment, or the name of the drug. General information about clinical trials is available from the NCI Web site, cancer.gov/clinicaltrials.

Advanced or recurrent colorectal cancer requires different treatments:

- **Metastatic colorectal cancer**: Colorectal cancer can spread to distant organs such as the liver, lungs, and ovaries. At this stage a combination

---

255   nci.nih.gov.

of surgery, radiation, and chemotherapy can slow the disease and sometimes shrink the tumor. However, it is rarely curable.

- **Metastatic colorectal cancer to the liver:**
  - Chemotherapy followed by resection
  - Radiofrequency ablation or cryosurgery
  - Clinical trials of hepatic chemoembolization with radiation therapy (for more specific results, refine the search by using other search features, such as the location of the trial, the type of treatment, or the name of the drug; see clinical trials above).

Talk to your doctor about a treatment option that works well for you.

Skin Cancer

There are three types of skin cancer, (1) basal cell carcinoma and (2) squamous cell carcinoma, which are referred to as nonmelanocytic skin cancers (NMSC), and (3) melanoma. More than 800,000 skin cancers are diagnosed each year. The NMSC are easily treatable and rarely metastasize. Melanomas are less common and deadly, accounting for more than eight thousand deaths annually.[1]

Risk Factors[256]

- Unprotected and/or excessive exposure to ultraviolet (UV) radiation
- Fair complexion
- Occupational exposures to coal tar, pitch, creosote, arsenic compounds, or radium
- Family history
- Multiple or atypical moles
- Severe sunburns as a child

Skin Cancer Symptoms

NMSC[1]

- An open sore that bleeds, oozes, or crusts and remains open for several weeks
- A reddish, raised patch or irritated area that may crust or itch, but rarely hurts

---

256   cancer.org/docroot/PED/content/ped_7_1_What_You_Need_To_Know_
    About_Skin_Cancer.asp?sitearea=&level= .

- A shiny pink, red, pearly white or translucent bump
- A pink growth with an elevated border and crusted central indentation
- A scar-like, white, yellow, or waxy area, often with a poorly defined border

Squamous Cell Cancer

Can often crust and bleed and appears as:
- A wart-like growth
- A persistent, scaly red patch with irregular borders that may bleed easily
- An open sore that persists for weeks
- An elevated growth with a rough surface and a central depression

Melanoma[257]

- A new, possibly large, irregularly shaped dark brownish spot with darker or black areas
- A simple mole that changes in color (particularly turning darker), size (growing), or texture (becoming firmer), and/or flakes or bleeds
- A lesion with an irregular border and red, white, blue, gray, or bluish-black areas or spots
- Shiny, firm, dome-shaped bumps anywhere on the body
- Dark lesions under the fingernails or toenails, on the palms, soles, tips of fingers and toes, or on mucous membranes (skin that lines the mouth, nose, vagina, and anus)

Skin Cancer Screening[258]

It is important for people forty and older to have annual skin screenings by a board-certified dermatologist. More frequent screenings are recommended if you are at high risk. Such high-risk people include those with a family history of skin cancer, those who are fair-skinned, those who have a history of severe sunburns when they were young, and those who live in southern regions of the United States. If you see any suspicious moles or new moles, see your doctor immediately.

---

257   cancer.net/patient/Cancer+Types/Melanoma.
258   mayoclinic.com/health/melanoma/DS00439/DSECTION=tests-and-di-agnosis.

Diagnosis

The only accurate way to diagnose skin cancer is by biopsy. Your dermatologist removes the suspicious growth or mole and sends it to a pathologist for examination.

If you are diagnosed with melanoma, the tumor will have to be staged to determine the extent of its growth. If you're diagnosed with melanoma, get a *second opinion* from a pathologist who is an expert in cancers of the skin. These subspecialists are called dermatopathologists. Your primary care physician or dermatologist should be able to direct you to one. Otherwise, you can find one at most medical schools or at a Designated Cancer Center near you. [259] NMSC are treated by excisional biopsy in the doctor's office.

Treatment[260]

If the melanoma has not spread beyond the skin, it is excised along with skin bordering the tumor. If the tumor has spread beyond the skin, the following treatments may be recommended:

- Surgical removal
- Chemotherapy
- Radiation therapy
- Biological therapy

Talk to your doctor about a treatment option that will work well for you.

Skin Cancer Prevention

Use sun screens and sun blockers that prevent both ultraviolet A and ultraviolet B exposure to prevent nonmelanocytic skin cancers (basal cell and squamous cell carcinomas—NMSC); sunscreens alone may not prevent melanomas, which also depends upon the *amount of time spent in the sun*. The higher the SPF (sun protection factor) written on the bottle of sunscreen, the better the protection; it does not mean the longer you can stay in the sun.[261] The best protection is to stay out of the sun.

---

259 Nci.nih.gov.

260 mayoclinic.com/health/melanoma/DS00439/DSECTION=treatments-and-drugs.

261 healthlink.mcw.edu/article/964647970.html.

> **Stay away from tanning salons—these prematurely age the skin and can cause skin cancer.**

See The ABCDs of Skin Cancer for more information about changes in the skin that you should be aware of.[262]

Prostate Cancer[263]

The American Cancer Society estimates 192,000 new cases and 27,000 deaths from prostate cancer in the United States for 2009, making prostate cancer the most common type of cancer found in American men. Prostate cancer is the second leading cause of cancer death in men.

One man in six will get prostate cancer during his lifetime, and 1 man in 35 will die of this disease. More than two million men in the United States who have had prostate cancer at some point are still alive today. The death rate for prostate cancer is going down, and the disease is being found earlier as well.[264]

Risk Factors/Prevention of Prostate Cancer

- Old age—over 70 percent of deaths from prostate cancer occur in men older than seventy-one.
- Race/ethnicity—African Americans are at a higher risk for developing prostate cancer and at an earlier age than white men.
- Family history of prostate cancer.
- Cigarette smoking.
- Obesity.
- High levels of testosterone.

Symptoms of Prostate Cancer

There may not be any symptoms associated with prostate cancer. None of the following symptoms are specific for cancer; they may be seen in a benign condition called benign prostatic hypertrophy (BPH) or enlargement of the prostate. Some of these include:

---

262   nasdonline.org/docs/d001201-d001300/d001207/d001207.html.
263   cancer.net/patient/Cancer+Types/Prostate+Cancer.
264   cancer.org/docroot/CRI/content/CRI_2_2_1X_How_many_men_get_ prostate_cancer_36.asp?sitearea=.

- Frequent urination
- Weak or interrupted urine flow
- Hematuria (blood in the urine)
- The urge to urinate frequently at night

If you find blood in your semen or experience pain or burning during urination, see your doctor immediately for further testing.

If cancer has spread beyond the prostate gland, you may experience

- Pain in the back, hips, thighs, shoulders, or other bones
- Unexplained weight loss
- Fatigue

Other symptoms may develop depending on the location of the metastasized tumor.

Prostate Cancer Screening

Currently, there are no specific tests to screen for prostate cancer. The tests used now, a blood test that measures PSA levels and a digital rectal exam (DRE), have low sensitivity and specificity (30 to 40 percent). For example, three out of four men with an elevated PSA (greater than 4.0 ng/ml) do not have prostate cancer, and one out of three men with a normal PSA has prostate cancer. If you have a family history of prostate cancer or are African American, you should be screened annually beginning at the age of forty-five; otherwise, begin annual screening at age fifty after weighing the pros and cons of screening with your doctor.

Note: Because of the low specificity of the screening tests, there is considerable controversy regarding screening. Recently a report was released by the Task Force that recommended men over seventy-five not be screened for prostate cancer. For men younger than age seventy-five, the benefits of screening for prostate cancer were uncertain and the balance of benefits and harms could not be determined.[265] The reason for this uncertainty is that a positive PSA means that you must have a biopsy done to determine if there is cancer. Prostate cancer grows so slowly that even if the biopsy is positive, it is unlikely that the tumor will kill you, even if you do nothing else. A recent clinical trial found no evidence that PSA screening of asymptomatic

---

265   USPSTF "Screening for prostate cancer: U.S. Preventive Services Task Force Recommendations Statement." Annals of Internal Medicine 149: 185, 2008.

men decreased the risk of dying from prostate cancer.[266] In another trial, they found that forty-eight men had to be treated for prostate cancer to save one from dying from the disease.[267] Since the tumor grows so slowly, if it is localized to the prostate gland, many doctors are recommending watchful waiting (see below).

If you're diagnosed with prostate cancer, get a *second opinion* from a pathologist who is an expert in prostate cancer. Contact a Designated Cancer Center for the name of an expert.[268]

Prostate Cancer Treatment[269]

There are various treatment options for prostate cancer. To determine the option that's right for you, you and your doctor should take into account the following:

- Your age and life expectancy
- Any other serious health problems you may have
- The stage and grade of your cancer
- Your feelings (and your doctor's opinion) about the need to treat the cancer
- The chance that each type of treatment will cure your cancer (or provide some other measure of benefit)
- Your feelings about the side effects common with each treatment

Numerous studies have suggested that men with prostate cancer face a different problem from other types of cancers—too much treatment, which wastes resources and money and needlessly subjects men to the pain and risks of surgery or radiation. Talk to your doctor about a treatment that works well for you.

1. *Watchful Waiting (or expectant management)*

---

266   G. L. Andriole, et al. "Mortality Results from a Randomized Prostate-Cancer Screening Trial," *NEJM* 360:1310, 2009.

267   F. H. Schroeder, et al. "Screening and Prostate-Cancer Mortality in a Randomized European Study," *NEJM* 360:1320, 2009.

268   nci.nih.gov.

269   cancer.org/docroot/CRI/content/CRI_2_2_4X_How_Is_Prostate_Cancer_Treated_36.asp?sitearea=.

Because prostate cancer often grows so slowly, some men may never need treatment for their cancer. Instead, their doctor may suggest an approach called "watchful waiting" (also called expectant management).

This approach involves closely watching the cancer (with PSA testing) without using treatment such as surgery or radiation therapy. It may be a good option if the cancer is not causing any symptoms, will probably grow slowly, and is small and contained in one place in the prostate.

2. *Surgery*

The name for removing the prostate is radical prostatectomy. The urologist's expertise is crucial for prostate cancer treatment. A study published recently in *The Journal of the National Cancer Institute* found that the cancer was less likely to come back in patients whose doctors had performed 250 or more operations.[270] Their recurrence rate was 10.7 percent, compared with 17.9 percent in men whose doctors had performed fewer prostatectomies.

3. *External Beam Radiation*

This treatment uses beams of high-energy X-rays or particles to kill cancer cells.[271]

4. *Radioactive Seed Implants (brachytherapy)*

Radioactive seeds are implanted directly into the prostate. The seeds deliver a higher dose of radiation than do external beams, but over a substantially longer period of time. The therapy is generally used in men with small to medium lower-grade cancers.[2]

5. *Hormonal Therapy*

Androgen ablation or androgen-deprivation therapy is used to reduce the amount of testosterone in the blood. Side effects include erectile dysfunction.

Side Effects of Prostate Cancer Treatment

The Task Force found convincing evidence that treatment for prostate cancer detected by screening causes moderate to substantial harms such as erectile dysfunction, urinary incontinence, bowel dysfunction, and death. Thus, the

---

270　　[1]Denise Grady in the NY Times, "Cancer Patients Lost in a Maze of Uneven Care" July 29, 2007.

271　　http://mayoclinic.com/health/radiation-therapy/MY00299.

Task Force recommends that the physician discuss the potential benefits and harms of screening with the patient. [272]

Lung Cancer

Lung cancer is the number-one cancer killer, and tobacco smoke is responsible for 87 percent of lung cancers. If everyone quit smoking 200,000 lung cancer deaths and another 200,000 deaths from other cancers, cardiovascular disease, and chronic lung disease would be prevented every year.[273] Passive smoking, radon gas, and asbestos can also cause lung cancer.

Risk Factors for Lung Cancer

Active and passive smoking increases the risk of developing non-small cell lung cancer, the most common form of lung cancer.

Symptoms of Lung Cancer

- Fatigue
- Cough
- Shortness of breath
- Chest pain, if a tumor invades a structure within the chest or involves the lining of the lung
- Loss of appetite
- Coughing up phlegm or mucus
- Hemoptysis (coughing up blood)

Lung Cancer Diagnosis

Screening for lung cancer is not recommended. If you have symptoms suggestive of lung cancer, your doctor must find out whether it's from cancer or something else. Your doctor may ask about your personal and family medical history. There are various tests and procedures to perform to diagnose lung cancer. If you are diagnosed with lung cancer, get a *second opinion* before beginning treatment. Contact a Designated Cancer Center for information about second opinions. [274]

---

272   USPSTF "Screening for prostate cancer: U.S. Preventive Services Task Force Recommendations Statement." Annals of Internal Medicine 149: 185, 2008.

273   cancer.org/docroot/PED/content/PED_10_2X_Cigarette_Smoking_and_Cancer.asp.

274   nci.nih.gov.

Chapter 12

Take Control of Chronic Obstructive Pulmonary Disease (COPD)

Objectives
- Recognize the symptoms of COPD
- Recognize the risks of COPD
- Understand how to treat COPD
- Some tips to help you manage COPD

Actual case: Taken from the *NY Times*, November 29, 2007 "From Smoking Boom, a Major Killer of Women," by Denise Grady.

For Jane, a fifty-nine-year-old president of a small company, the crisis came five years ago when she got up to go to work she could barely breathe. Although she quit smoking ten years earlier, the damage was already done after thirty years of smoking. After several days in the hospital she was sent home tethered to an oxygen tank, and a pocketful of prescriptions. Jane had COPD, which is a chronic progressive disease that permanently damages the lungs and most often caused by smoking. It used to be an old man's disease, but because of the increase in the number of women smoking the death rate in women has tripled from 1980 to 2000 and more women have died or been hospitalized from the disease than men. *If everyone in America stopped smoking today, the*

Myth: Once I quit smoking, my COPD will go away.
Fact: Lung damage caused by cigarette smoking is permanent. It won't go away.

Definition

COPD is the fourth leading cause of death in the United States, killing 120,000 Americans each year. About 12 million Americans are known to have it, and 12 million more cases have not been diagnosed. Half the patients are under sixty-five years of age, and the disease has left approximately 900,000 Americans too debilitated to work. Medical bills and lost productivity amount to $42 billion a year. COPD actually comprises two illnesses: emphysema and chronic bronchitis. Emphysema destroys the air sacs in the lung, while chronic bronchitis causes inflammation, congestion, and scarring in the airways. [275]

COPD is so unrecognized by the public that researches say the "O" in COPD should stand for "obscure." COPD is misdiagnosed, neglected, improperly treated, and stigmatized as self-induced, often creating a lot of guilt among victims who are smokers. It is commonly mistaken for asthma, especially in women, and treated with the wrong drugs.

Doctors sometimes prescribe similar medications for COPD and asthma even though the appropriate treatments differ. The first-line maintenance therapy for most patients with asthma is an inhaled corticosteroid, with the addition of a bronchodilator, if needed, to control symptoms. However, the reverse is true for the treatment of COPD. Bronchodilators are the first-line maintenance treatment for COPD. Treatment with inhaled corticosteroids is reserved only for selected patients whose COPD is not adequately managed with bronchodilators. [276]

Table 12.1 Differences between COPD and asthma

COPD	Asthma
Smoking history	Passive smoking is a risk factor
Onset in midlife	Onset early in life
Symptoms often consistent from day to day	Symptoms episodic and vary from day to day
Breath sounds may include wheezing	Breath sounds may include wheezing

275   nytimes.com/2007/11/29/health/29lung.html.
276   aarc.org/klein/what_is_copd.asp.

Increased risk of osteoporosis, cardiovascular disease, and diabetes	Allergy, rhinitis (runny nose), and/or eczema present
Airflow limitation partially reversible	Airflow limitation largely reversible
Family history not a predictor	Family history usually a predictor
Hyperinflation may be present	Hyperinflation usually not present

Source: Boehringer Ingelheim Pharmaceuticals, Inc. or its affiliated companies, 2009. All Rights Reserved.

Risk Factors

- Smoking is the primary cause of COPD. It is ten times more likely that a smoker will get COPD than a nonsmoker.
- Being exposed to cigarette smoke (passive smoking) can increase your risk of COPD.
- Exposure to indoor or outdoor pollutants can cause COPD. If your job exposes you to toxic chemicals or pollutants, you will also have an increased risk of developing COPD. A recent study found that an estimated 19.2 percent of COPD cases can be caused by a rare genetic condition called alpha-1 antitrypsin deficiency.

Symptoms of COPD[277]

Even the slightest activity (such as walking to the mailbox) leaves you short of breath. It is often described as "breathing through a straw." You may cough up mucus or phlegm. The disease gradually progresses because of the large capacity of the lungs. People often adjust psychologically, cutting back on some activities and attributing their symptoms of shortness of breath as being out of shape or getting old.

If you're a smoker, be sure your doctor performs a breathing test (spirometry). The disease is not curable but it is treatable if diagnosed early.

Diagnosis of COPD[278]

a. History and physical exam
   i. Patients are usually current or past smokers over the age of forty with a history of shortness of breath upon physical exertion and a chronic productive cough.

---

277   copdguide.com/copd-is-different.asp.
278   pulmonologychannel.com/copd/diagnosis.shtml.

ii. The physical exam may show barrel chest, decreased breath sounds, and wheezing.
b. Pulmonary function tests, to confirm or support diagnosis of COPD
c. Oximetry measures oxygenation of blood
d. Radiological procedures
e. Arterial blood gases
f. Measure alpha-1-antitrypsin levels in blood if a person is suspected of having a genetic deficiency of this protein

Under-diagnosis of COPD [1, 2]

- COPD symptoms are often mistaken for "getting older."
- COPD is easily confused with asthma.
- COPD symptoms are often misunderstood in its early stages.
- People think that if they quit smoking the coughing and breathlessness will go away. These symptoms are signs of a serious disease and you should seek medical attention right away.

Preventing COPD [1, 2]

- Quit smoking
- Exercise regularly
- Eat a healthy diet
- Avoid triggers of COPD
    o Some people find hot humid air makes it harder to breathe.
    o Some people find cold air makes it harder to breathe.
    o COPD can be treated at any stage of the disease.

Health Risks Associated with COPD

- Osteoporosis, weakened muscles, and cataracts from overprescribed steroids, such as prednisone, used to treat the disease
- Heart disease
- Hypertension
- Lung cancer

Treatment Options[279]

Many patients and doctors mistakenly think little can be done for COPD. Although it is incurable, it is treatable. These treatment options could help you lead a better and longer life. Talk to your doctor about the treatment options that are best for you.

- Drugs
    - Inhalers to open airways and quell inflammation
        - Maintenance inhalers
- Taken every day to maintain control of your COPD
- Work gradually and lasts four to twenty-four hours
- Must be taken every day for full effect
        - Rescue inhalers
- Taken in times of emergencies to help you catch your breath when symptoms suddenly get worse.
- Works quickly and lasts four to six hours.
    - Antibiotics to fight lung infection
    - Vaccines to prevent flu and pneumonia
- Pulmonary rehabilitation (special breathing techniques to make the most of their diminished lungs)
- Education about the disease (programs are not available across the country)
- Preventive measures, especially quitting smoking
- Exercise programs
- Oxygen
- Lung surgery

---

279   copdguide.com/treatment-options.jsp.

Chapter 13

Take Control of Dementia

Objectives:
- To be aware of the warning signs of dementia
- To understand the risk factors for Alzheimer's disease
- To understand how to slow the progression of Alzheimer's disease
- To provide you with care giving information for loved ones with dementia

Some personal and clinical experiences: Although there are many illnesses that families deal with, Alzheimer's disease is perhaps the most difficult. One reason is the strong resistance and denial of the disease by those affected and their families. It is all too common for the patient or spouse to refuse to accept that they or a loved one is experiencing signs of dementia.

Actual case: Recently, a forty-two-year-old male patient of mine (L. K.) came into session and said how concerned he was about his seventy-seven-year-old mother, whom he found to be forgetful lately. He stated that when he expressed his concerns to his father, he was told "there was nothing to be concerned about." After several more experiences of his mother's forgetfulness, he strongly encouraged his father to set up an appointment with their doctor. Once again, his father dismissed his concerns and refused to follow up. My patient wanted advice from me as to where to go from here in order to get his mother evaluated. Unfortunately, there was little I could offer, as denial of this disease is all too common. I suggested he continue to confront his father and also talk to his mother, who he feared would be more difficult than his father. As of this date, both of his parents refuse to see a doctor.

Alzheimer's disease is the most common form of dementia, a general term for the loss of memory and other intellectual abilities serious enough to interfere with daily life. Alzheimer's disease accounts for 50 to 70 percent of dementia cases. Five million Americans have been diagnosed, and there were 360,000 new cases diagnosed in 2009. Seventy percent of people with Alzheimer's and other dementias live at home and are frequent users of home- and community-based services for help with activities of daily living. In 2005, people with Alzheimer's or other dementias incurred $21 billion in state and federal Medicaid costs and $91 billion in Medicare costs to cover nursing home costs.[280] Although there is presently no cure for Alzheimer's, there are treatments for symptoms. These treatments, combined with the right services and support, allows Americans living with Alzheimer's to have better lives. There is an accelerating worldwide effort under way to find better ways to treat the disease, delay its onset, or prevent it from developing.

The phrase "sandwich generation" has been used to describe those adults, roughly forty to fifty years old, who not only care for their own children but are in the position of caring for or making health care decisions for ill parents. The patient I referred to above fits into this category, as he has two children, ages two and four, and will soon be in a position of helping his parents as the illness progresses.

The emotional toll of watching a loved one progress into an illness such as Alzheimer's, along with the stress of having to make serious healthcare choices, can be overwhelming. In most healthcare situations, people are faced with illnesses that can be "understood." Cancer, heart attacks, and diabetes are among a wide variety of health problems that often have clear-cut diagnoses and treatments. Patients and or loved ones come together to offer support and understanding, which makes the treatment process linear and focused. Unfortunately, all too often the emotional denial of Alzheimer's adds another dimension to an already difficult situation. Since early diagnosis and treatment is essential, the time delay that occurs between the first symptoms and acute onset is a major concern.

One early symptom of Alzheimer's is anger. The patient can often be experienced by family members as hostile, which adds to the fear loved ones have to confront the issues. People often feel punished for trying to help and back off out of their own fear of rejection. The emotional aspects of Alzheimer's affect all who are concerned, often times more than the patient themselves.

In our practice (Joan and I), we have seen siblings fighting with each other, sons and daughters angry with their parents, and serious family dysfunction arise out of the stress of this disease. Often, family members simply give up and wait until the disease is so pronounced that denial is impossible.

---

280   Alz.org.

My two brothers and I experienced Alzheimer's firsthand, as our mother first showed early symptoms at the age of seventy-five. Our eighty-one-year-old father refused to acknowledge Mom's early symptoms, even though we consistently pointed out her memory decline, depression, and anxiety. It was not until our father passed away, at the age of eighty-three, that we were able to take control and get our mother the medical attention she required. Unfortunately, her illness progressed quickly, and she passed away just two months shy of her eightieth birthday. Had treatment begun earlier, perhaps we could have slowed the progress of this disease.

In today's world of strict medical confidentiality, it becomes even more difficult for family members to have contact or updates from their parents' physicians without a signed consent. This can further complicate the free flow of important information that family members can offer to the treating physician. One of the few choices families have is to conduct an "intervention," which consists of family members sitting down with the parents and confronting the issue directly. Hopefully, with numbers comes influence, and progress may be achieved.

Emotional Impact on the Care Givers

Dealing with Alzheimer's as a caregiver is extremely draining emotionally, and it is imperative that caregivers talk openly about the stress, sadness, anxiety, and other feelings Alzheimer's can bring out. Support groups, therapy, and friends can offer emotional comfort and be a source of stress release. Although many believe they can or should be able to handle it alone, rarely is this a good strategy. When dealing with a disease that leaves people feeling so out of control, reaching out to others cannot be stressed enough. In my own experience with my mother, talking daily to my wife, Joan (who is also a psychotherapist) was extremely helpful. Without her constant support, I don't think I could have gotten through it. Talking to my brothers, kids, friends, and co-workers was also tremendously helpful.

We all hope Alzheimer's will never affect anyone we love; however, tens of thousands each year will be diagnosed with this disease. It is our responsibility to recognize the physical aspects of this disease as well as the emotional toll it can take on us all.

Myths about Alzheimer's:

Myth: You have to be older than sixty-five to get Alzheimer's disease.

Fact: More than 10 percent of the people suffering from Alzheimer's are under sixty-five; you can begin to show signs in your thirties.[281]

Myth: Memory loss is a natural part of aging and is nothing to be concerned about.

Fact: The extent of memory loss from Alzheimer's goes well beyond normal boundaries, as ultimately the person who is affected can no longer recognize who they're looking at in the mirror.

Definitions

- *Dementia* is the progressive decline in cognitive function due to damage or disease in the body beyond what might be expected from normal aging.
- *Alzheimer's disease* is the most common cause of dementia. It is a progressive, degenerative brain disease that affects memory, thinking, and behavior.

The rate of progression is different for each person, but generally, if Alzheimer's develops rapidly, it progresses rapidly, and if it develops slowly, it will progress slowly. As discussed in chapter 5, it is important for you to have thought about and prepared advanced directives, such as a living will, so if you are afflicted with this disease, you receive the care *you want*. in the absence of advanced directives, the doctors are obliged to do everything that is technologically available to prolong your life.

Risk Factors for Alzheimer's Disease [1,282,283]

- A family history of Alzheimer's disease
- Mutation of a specific gene
- Advanced age (Alzheimer's affects mostly older adults but can sometimes begin in younger individuals)
- Gender (women live longer than men so they are more likely to develop Alzheimer's)
- Hypertension
- History of head trauma
- Obesity
- Diabetes

---

281   Alz.org.
282   cnn.com/2009/HEALTH/01/26/health.calories.memory.
283   newswise.com/articles/view/539441/?sc=dwhr.

- High levels of homocysteine (a body chemical that may contribute to chronic disease)
- Depression

Symptoms of Alzheimer's Disease [284,285]

Although dementia is common in older adults, *it is not a normal consequence of aging.* About half of Americans with Alzheimer's disease are in the early stages of the disease, where certain interventions may sometimes slow its progression. The information below will help you recognize the early signs of the disease so you can get the help you need:

- Gradually increasing memory loss and memory impairment (must be present to diagnose dementia)
- Confusion
- Unclear thinking, including losing problem-solving skills
- Agitated behavior or delusions
- Becoming lost in formerly familiar circumstances
- Loss of interest in daily or usual activities
- Changes in personality
- Misplacing things

Diagnosing Alzheimer's Disease [1,2]

You should go to a geriatrician or neurologist if you suspect you have the symptoms of dementia. Geriatricians are internal medicine or family practice doctors who specialize in treating the elderly. Geriatricians also are trained in planning and implementing interventions for common geriatric syndromes such as dementia, delirium, drug misuse, depression, falls, incontinence, pressure ulcers, and functional decline. To find a geriatrician in your area, go to abms.org.

Call your healthcare provider if someone close to you experiences symptoms of dementia or if a person with this disorder experiences a sudden change in mental status (a rapid change may indicate another illness).

Alzheimer's disease usually has characteristic patterns of symptoms and can be diagnosed by an experienced physician.

---

284   Alz.org
285   health.nytimes.com/health/guides/disease/alzheimers-disease/overview. html?print=1.

Discuss the situation with your healthcare provider if you are caring for a person with this disorder and the condition deteriorates to the point where you can no longer care for the person in your home.

Find a gerontologist or neurologist to diagnose and treat your dementia. He or she will determine whether dementia is present by evaluating memory impairment along with changes in one of the following:

- Language
- Decision-making ability
- Judgment
- Attention
- And other areas of mental function and personality

The next step is to clarify the type of dementia. This is accomplished by taking a detailed patient history, performing a physical exam, including a neurological exam, and performing a mental status examination.

A careful evaluation by your doctor is important to look for *treatable causes* of dementias, such as:

- Thyroid disease
- Vitamin B12 or B9 deficiency
- Brain tumor
- Drug and medication toxicity
- Anemia
- Severe depression

Stages of Alzheimer's Disease [286, 287]

Alzheimer's is a progressive disease that is divided into four stages.

Signs of Early Stages

Symptoms may be subtle and mistaken for "natural aging." *Remember, dementia is not a normal part of aging.*

- Repeating statements
- Misplacing items
- Having trouble remembering names of things

286   Alz.org.
287   health.nytimes.com/health/guides/disease/alzheimers-disease/overview.html?print=1.

- Getting lost on familiar routes
- Personality changes
- Losing interest in things
- Difficulty in performing routine tasks like balancing a checkbook.

Signs of Moderate Stages

- Aphasia (loss of ability to use words)
- Apraxia (cannot perform activities that they are physically able and willing to do)
- Confusion
- Agitation
- Insomnia

Signs of Advanced Stages

- Forgetting details about current events
- Forgetting events in your own life history, unaware of who you are
- Problems choosing proper clothing
- Hallucinations, arguments, striking out, and violent behavior
- Delusions, depression, agitation
- Difficulty performing basic tasks like preparing meals and driving
- Will most likely need 24/7 nursing home care at this stage

End Stage

- Cannot understand language
- Cannot recognize family members
- Cannot perform basic tasks of daily living such as eating, dressing, and bathing
- Bedfast
- Dysphagia (difficulty swallowing)
- Intercurrent infections

Issues to Discuss with Your Doctor about Alzheimer's Disease:[288]

1. How can we be sure my symptoms aren't the result of a stroke, mental illness, or another treatable condition?

---

288   health.nytimes.com/health/guides/disease/alzheimers-disease/overview. html?print=1.

2. What stage of Alzheimer's disease am I in? What comes next?
3. What can I do to preserve my health and mental abilities for as long as possible?
4. What physical symptoms should I anticipate?
5. My children are worried about inheriting this illness. Would it be useful for our family to undergo genetic testing?
6. What drugs are currently available for Alzheimer's disease, and how well do they work?
7. My family is afraid to let me drive. Would you refer me for a driving evaluation so we can have an objective opinion of my ability?
8. What can I do to make things easier on my family?

Make sure you express your preferences for future care by using advanced directives, based on your values, not your caregiver's.

Preventive Measures[289,290,291]

Although there is no cure for Alzheimer's disease, here are some practices to incorporate into your lifestyle to reduce the risk of Alzheimer's:

- Eat fewer calories.
- Eat cold-water fish (like tuna, salmon, and mackerel) rich in omega-3 fatty acids, at least two to three times per week.
- Reduce your intake of linoleic acid found in margarine, butter, and dairy products.
- Increase antioxidants like carotenoids, vitamin E, and vitamin C by eating plenty of darkly colored fruits and vegetables.
- Control high blood pressure.
- Stay mentally and socially active throughout your life.
- Consider talking to your doctor about the risks and benefits of taking nonsteroidal anti-inflammatory drugs (NSAIDs) like ibuprofen (Advil, Motrin), sulindac (Clinoril), or indomethacin (Indocin) to delay the symptoms of Alzheimer's.
- Statin drugs, a class of medications normally used for high cholesterol, may help lower your risk of Alzheimer's disease. Discuss these with your doctor.

---

289   Alz.org.
290   newswise.com/articles/view/539441/?sc=dwhr.
291   cnn.com/2009/HEALTH/01/26/health.calories.memory.

Tips for Keeping the Brain Sharp[1,292]

A large national survey from the University of Michigan found that over a ten-year period ending in 2002, memory loss and thinking problems were down significantly among seniors aged seventy and older, from 12.2 percent to 8.7 percent. That's a change that translates into hundreds of thousands of men and women, though Alzheimer's is still a top concern for millions worldwide.

Researchers aren't sure why the decrease in cognitive impairment is occurring, but they suspect that the habits of a better educated and more affluent older generation, less likely to smoke and more likely to eat better and get regular exercise, may be helping to keep the brain young. Here are some general guidelines:

- *Stay mentally challenged*
- *Keep working*
- *Maintain an active social life.* Men and women who remained socially connected with friends and family as they aged had sharper memories, a study from the Harvard School of Public Health reported.
- *Exercise*
- *Keep your cholesterol in check.*
- *Control your blood pressure.*
- *Eat fish rich in omega-3 fatty acids.* Once again, research showed that eating oily fish like salmon, mackerel, and anchovies may help lower the risk of memory decline and stroke in healthy older adults. Fish that was baked or broiled, but not fried, appeared to benefit the brain.
- *Surf the Web.* Finally, searching the Internet may be good the brain. Researchers at the University of California, Los Angeles, found that surfing the Web triggers key centers in the brain involved in decision-making and complex reasoning and was better for the brain than reading a book.

---

292   health.nytimes.com/health/guides/disease/alzheimers-disease/overview.html?print=1.

Treatment of Alzheimer's [293,294]

There is no cure for Alzheimer's disease or vascular dementia. Rather, families and providers try to manage the disease. Treatments focus on the following:

- Slow the progression of the disease
- Manage behavioral problems, confusion, and agitation
- Modify the home environment
- Support family members and other caregivers

Lifestyle changes such as social interactions with a reliable companion may also help slow down the progression of the disease and increase communication skills. Some studies have suggested using bright-light therapy to reduce insomnia and wandering.[295] Listening to calming music may reduce wandering and restlessness and boost brain chemicals, ease anxiety, enhance sleep, and improve behavior. Pets have also been shown to relieve anxiety, as have regular massages, which are relaxing and provide social interactions.

In different stages of Alzheimer's, there may be physical or mental outbursts, general emotional distress, restlessness, pacing, yelling, hallucinations, and delusions. Recognize that the person is not purposely behaving inappropriately but is exhibiting further symptoms of the disease. Try to understand the cause and how symptoms relate to the disease. Changing the person's environment may make it easier to live with the disease. For example, removing obstacles and clutter in the house can help provide comfort and peace of mind.

Drug Approaches to Treat Alzheimer's Disease

Some prescription medications for cognitive symptoms:

293   Alz.org.
294   health.nytimes.com/health/guides/disease/alzheimers-disease/overview.
html?print=1.
295   aja.sagepub.com/cgi/content/abstract/15/1/18.

Table 13.1 Drugs used to treat Alzheimer's disease

Generic	Brand	Approved for	Side effects
Donepezil	Aricept	All stages	Nausea, vomiting, loss of appetite and increased frequency of bowel movements
Galantamine	Razadyne	Mild to moderate	Nausea, vomiting, loss of appetite and increased frequency of bowel movements
Memantine	Namenda	Moderate to severe	Headache, constipation, confusion and dizziness.
Rivastigmine	Exelon	Mild to moderate	Nausea, vomiting, loss of appetite and increased frequency of bowel movements
Tacrine	Cognex	Mild to moderate	Possible liver damage, nausea, and vomiting

Source: alz.org/alzheimers_disease_standard_prescriptions.asp

The three key drugs, Aricept, Razadyne, and Exelon, can interact with anti-cholinergic drugs, belladonna alkaloids, tri-cyclic antidepressants, first-generation antihistamines, many skeletal muscle relaxants, drugs for urinary incontinence, many antipsychotic drugs, and some anti-arrhythmic drugs.

Namenda is the newest drug and has benefited patients with moderately severe and severe Alzheimer's disease the most. Namenda is marketed for moderate-to-severe Alzheimer's, but a recent study suggests it is effective for all stages of the disease when used in combination with any one of the older Alzheimer's drugs.[296] Your doctor can help you decide which medication is right for you or your loved ones.

---

296   wsj.com/article/SB123603689949914421.html.

People with dementia are susceptible to serious side effects of antipsychotic drugs, including stroke and heart attack.

Sometimes these medications can cause an increase in the symptoms being treated. Risk and potential benefits of a drug should be carefully analyzed for any individual. The decision to use an antipsychotic drug needs to be considered with extreme caution. A recent analysis showed that atypical antipsychotics were associated with an increased risk of stroke and death in older adults with dementia. [297,298] The FDA has asked manufacturers to include a "black box" warning consumers and providers about the risks and a reminder that they are not approved to treat dementia symptoms. The warning states, "Elderly patients with dementia-related psychosis treated with atypical antipsychotic drugs (second generation drugs) are at an increased risk of death compared to placebo."

Antipsychotic medications that may cause hallucinations, delusions, aggression, agitation, hostility, and uncooperativeness include

- Aripiprazole (Abilify)
- Clozapine (Clozaril)
- Olanzapine (Zyprexa)
- Quetiapine (Seroquel)
- Risperidone (Risperdal)
- Ziprasidone (Geodon)

Pharmacists are the medication experts on the healthcare team and play a unique role in working with patients and providers to ensure that drugs are safely prescribed. Talk to your pharmacist about any black box warnings on your or your loved one's medications.

Individuals with dementia should only use these antipsychotic drugs when,

- Their behavioral symptoms are due to mania or psychosis
- The symptoms present a danger to others
- The patient is experiencing inconsolable or persistent distress, a significant decline in function or substantial difficulty receiving needed care

---

297   L.S. Schneider, et al., "Effectiveness of Atypical Antipsychotic Drugs in Patients with Alzheimer's Disease," *NEJM* 355: 1505, 2006.
298   msnbc.msn.com/id/15223481/.

Antipsychotic medications should not be used to sedate or restrain persons with dementia. If these drugs must be used, the minimum dosage should be used for the minimum amount of time possible. Adverse side effects require careful monitoring.

Care facilities, such as assisted nursing facilities and nursing homes, are required by law to employ or obtain the services of a licensed pharmacist who provides consultation on all aspects of the provision of pharmacy services in the facility and helps to identify, evaluate, and address pharmaceutical concerns that affect resident care, medical care, or quality of life issues.

Dietary supplements are reported to be helpful for Alzheimer's patients. These include two of the B vitamins—vitamin B9 and vitamin B12—while antioxidants like vitamin E are also reported to be helpful. *Ginko biloba* is supposed to increase circulation and is often considered helpful for the disease. Talk to your doctor before taking any dietary supplements! They may also interfere with medications or make you more prone to bleeding.

Some questions to ask the doctor about prescription medications you or your loved ones are taking for Alzheimer's:

- What kind of assessment will you use to determine if the drug is effective?
- How much time will pass before you will be able to assess the drug's effectiveness?
- How will you monitor for possible side effects?
- What effects should we watch for at home? When should we call you?
- Is one treatment option more likely than another to interfere with medications for other conditions?
- What are the concerns with stopping one drug treatment and beginning another?
- At what stage of the disease would you consider it appropriate to stop using the drug?

Prognosis[299]

The prognosis is poor. This condition usually progresses steadily and total disability is common. Death normally occurs within fifteen years, usually from an infection or a failure of other body systems.

---

299   Ninds.nih.gov.

Possible Complications of Alzheimer's Disease [1, 2]

As the disease progresses, the patient with Alzheimer's is no longer able to function or care for herself. She will also be prone to many of the following complications:

- Bedsores, loss of ability to move joints, infections (urinary tract and pneumonia)
- Complications due to immobility due to end stages of disease
- Falls and broken bones
- Loss of ability to interact with others
- Malnutrition and dehydration
- Failure of organ systems
- Harmful or violent behavior to oneself or others
- Side effects of medications

Caregiving for the Alzheimer's Patient

Setting Up Home Care[300,301]

Soon after diagnosis of Alzheimer's, it will be necessary to make some changes to help provide a sense of well being and physical safety for your loved one.

Try to encourage and maintain the independence of the person for as long as possible. To help maintain that independence, there is a technique called graded assistance combined with practice (as in "practice makes perfect") and positive reinforcement. Graded assistance is helping the person with the least amount of aid necessary to accomplish a task. Dementia therapy has been used with some success with people with Alzheimer's. This type of therapy includes playing your loved one's favorite type of music to help alleviate aggression and agitation, especially during mealtimes and bath. Other types of therapy that have been shown to help calm patients include a pet companion, lighting manipulation, art, and group therapies that concentrate on cognitive skills and social activities.

Also, try to adjust your communication style to the patient's changing needs as the disease progresses. Remember, in the early stages of the disease you will be communicating with a loved one that may be in denial compared

---

300   helpguide.org/elder/alzheimers_disease_dementias_caring_caregivers.htm.
301   Alz.org/national/documents/book_coachbroylesplaybook.pdf.

to the middle stages of the disease when they may be aggressive or paranoid, or the later stages of the disease, when they may be dying. For advice, support, or information about Alzheimer's disease call the Alzheimer's hotline (1- 800- 272-3900).

Remember to be sensitive and gentle about informing loved ones of the diagnosis. Try to have a positive attitude, and learn how to communicate with the Alzheimer's patient. For example, don't argue or try to change the person's mind, even if you believe your request is rational. This behavior is part of the disease process. Try not to take behavior problems personally. When you have to manage behavioral problems, be patient, kind, flexible, supportive, and calm. The disease is no one's fault. Accept the symptoms of the disease and proceed from there. Warm, supportive care is essential to the loved one's well being as well as the person's sense of worth.

In addition:

- Schedule all visitors to avoid surprises.
- Establish routines in activities of daily living (the things we do in normal living such as feeding ourselves, bathing, dressing, and grooming).
- Maintain social contacts and fun.
- Set up a safe home environment.
- Consider transferring to a facility if care giving becomes unmanageable at home.
- Join an Alzheimer's support group to get emotional support for yourself.
- Be sure you enroll your loved one in the Safe Return Program implemented by the Alzheimer's Association, which requires that a person with Alzheimer's disease wear an ID bracelet to help find them if they wander off.

Many caregivers ask, when will I know that it's not safe to leave my loved one alone in the house for more than a few minutes? Here are some answers:

- When they forget to turn off the oven or stove
- When they forget to close the front door
- When they cannot use the phone to call for help
- When they do not notice dangerous situations, such as a fire
- When they are unpredictable or confused under stressful conditions
- When they wander or become disoriented

- When they do not realize when they need supervision for some activities

If you are living with an Alzheimer's patient, try hiring a home aide for a few hours a day to give you time for yourself or find an adult day care center near you to drop off your loved one for a day.[302,303,304]

Keep Careful Medical Records

To ensure proper communication and coordination of care with healthcare providers, keep a notebook to record each doctor's visit and lab and X-ray results, along with medications. You will be taking your loved one back and forth to doctors and hospitals, and having this information at your fingertips will keep them safe and ensure they get the right care.

Care Giving Tasks

Eighty percent of long term care in the USA is provided by family members and friends. For helpful tips on care giving, download *Coach Broyles Playbook for Alzheimer's Caregiving*. Coach Broyles is the athletic director at the University of Arkansas and gives valuable tips from personal experience.[305]

These tips depend on the needs of the person, which change as the dementia progresses:

- Shopping for groceries, preparing meals, and providing transportation
- Helping the patient keep track of the medications they are taking
- Managing their finances and legal affairs
- Supervising the person to avoid unsafe activities, such as wandering and getting lost
- Bathing, dressing, feeding, helping the person use the toilet, or providing incontinence care
- Making arrangements for medical care and in-home aid or in-home healthcare, assisted living, or nursing home care[306]

---

302 Niapublications.org/pubs/long-distance/So_Far)Away_Twenty_Questions_For_Long_Distance_Caregivers.pdf.
303 helpguide.org/elder/alzheimers_disease_dementias_caring_caregivers.htm.
304 Benefitscheckup.org.
305 Alz.org/national/documents/book_coachbroylesplaybook.pdf.
306 Alz.washington.edu.

In addition to providing for a person's physical needs for safety, nutrition, and good health, there is a full range of personal and emotional needs:

- Provide companionship
- Provide stimulation
- Increase self-esteem
- Make them feel valued
- Treat them with dignity and respect

Taking Care of the Care Giver [307,308]

If you are calmer and "in control" in stressful situations, you will feel better and so will everyone around you, including your loved one with Alzheimer's. Please try to take care of your emotional wellbeing, because it is common to experience high levels of stress and depression when care giving. One study found that in the year before their loved one's death, half of the care givers spent at least forty-six hours a week assisting the person with dementia, which results in a lot of stress. There are counseling and support programs for care givers that can help you reduce your level of stress and, as a result, delay your loved one's placement in a nursing home (for more on this topic, see chapter 14, "How Our Emotions Affect Our Health"). Seek support groups and check out adult daycare facilities (similar to "mother's day out"), so you can have some time for yourself.

The care giver's experience affects many aspects of their lives. For example, care givers are more likely to report that their health is fair or poorer than that of non-caregivers. They also report more absences from work and fewer hours of work outside the home than non-care givers. Forty-nine percent of unpaid care givers of people with dementia had out-of-pocket care giving expenses that averaged $219 a month (for home aides).

Long-distance Care Giving

Ten percent of the 9.8 million care givers live more than two hours away from the person. We would suggest that you hire a *geriatric care manager* to help you manage your loved one's care from a distance. A geriatric care manager[309] is a licensed professional who assesses your loved one's ability to live independently in a home environment, develops an appropriate

---

307   Alz.org.
308   Benefitscheckup.org.
309   caremanager.org.

care plan for services and equipment, and organizes needed home services. Importantly, a geriatric care manager can continuously monitor your loved one for changes in their condition so the services they require can be altered to fit the circumstances.

The Best Facilities for Alzheimer's Patients [310,311,312,313]

Those facilities that specialize in treating Alzheimer's patients tend to be very expensive. If they are out of your price range, here are some criteria to look for in a general long-term care facility:

- Care givers help patients get out of bed.
- Care givers appear to enjoy what they do.
- Care givers interact with patients in their own language.
- Patients with dementia live together.
- The facility is generally safe and is located within in your area[314]

The National Institute on Aging has set up and financed Alzheimer's Disease Centers for patients and families affected by the disease: [1-5]

Diagnosis and medical management (costs may vary—centers may accept Medicare, Medicaid, and private insurance). Check with the center and Medicare. Although there is no cure for Alzheimer's, research has uncovered many treatments that delay the progression or help with its symptoms. There are many information sources on the Internet. Remember, being a care giver for this disease does not mean you are alone. Use the many resources available.

Answers to Commonly Asked Questions about Alzheimer's Disease:[315]

---

310   Eldercare.gov/Eldercare.NET/Public/Network/Network/aspx.
311   Helpguide.org.
312   Gilbertguide.com.
313   aahsa.org.
314   medicare.gov/NHCompare/Include/DataSection/Questions/SearchCriteria.asp?version=default&browser=Firefox percent7C2 percent7CWindows+Vista&language=English&defaultstatus=0&pagelist=Home&CookiesEnabledStatus=True.
315   health.nytimes.com/ref/health/healthguide/esn-alzheimers-ess.

I believe my wife has Alzheimer's disease. She is sensitive about her memory lapses. How can I get her to see her doctor?
Suggest she go for an annual exam or call the doctor's office and explain the situation. Suggest they call her to remind her about having an annual exam.

Am I at increased risk for Alzheimer's disease if my mother died with the disease?
Five to ten percent of Alzheimer's cases have a genetic link. Early onset Alzheimer's often runs in families. Late onset is the most common form of the disease and occurs in people sixty and older. It is not thought to run in families.

What does it mean to be in the middle stages of Alzheimer's?
The process of Alzheimer's disease can be described as a series of stages. Staging Alzheimer's disease gives people with the disease, their loved ones, and doctors and care givers a general guide to the pattern of the disease. This can help them make care decisions throughout the course of the disease. There is no clear line between the stages, and they may overlap.

Does a person die from Alzheimer's disease?
Alzheimer's disease is a progressive, degenerative disease of the brain where brain cells continue to die over time. People usually die of secondary infections, such as pneumonia.

Can the family doctor diagnose Alzheimer's disease?
A comprehensive assessment needs to be done by a trained physician for the diagnosis of Alzheimer's disease to be made. The person's family doctor may be able to do this assessment. Or she may refer to a memory clinic or specialist, such as a geriatrician or neurologist. Visit the Web site of the Alzheimer's Association to find professionals in your area.[316]

Can depression bring on symptoms like Alzheimer's disease?
Depression can have symptoms similar to Alzheimer's disease. It is important to see a doctor if any symptoms are present, because often times a condition, such as depression, can be treated.

Can people in their forties get Alzheimer's disease?
While most people get Alzheimer's disease after age sixty, early onset Alzheimer's disease can occur in one's forties.

---

316   Alz.org.

Chapter 14

How Our Emotions Affect Our Health

Objectives:
- To better understand our emotions
- To identify and accept the effects our emotions have on our physical health
- To deal with our emotions in a manner that will not negatively impact our illness but rather accelerate our recovery
- To communicate our emotions effectively to our loved ones and caregivers.

Stress, anxiety, anger, depression, and frustration are just some of the emotions that often go unidentified and untreated, especially when the primary focus is on physical illnesses. Individuals and their loved ones experiencing illness often find themselves feeling a general sense of anxiety, an "uneasiness" that may be pervasive on a daily basis. For the individual going through a serious illness, untreated emotional issues can negatively affect the course and outcome of treatment.

These underlying feelings can lead couples to experience marital conflict, displace anger toward children or parents, and cause other dysfunctional reactions within the family. It is extremely important that if any of these conflicts arise, they be dealt with in a professional setting, with a trained therapist. Left untreated, these conflicts can undermine the recovery process.

In this section, we will talk about six rules for managing emotions.

Rule Number 1: Express Your Feelings Appropriately

Case 1: A couple came in for marriage counseling. The husband was a forty-three-year-old attorney, and his wife was a forty-one-year-old nurse/homemaker. They had two sons, ages ten and twelve. The husband was honest when he acknowledged that the only reason he agreed to counseling was because his wife had been "relentless" about it. She stated, two years ago, her husband was diagnosed with diabetes, and since then she had experienced him as moody, short tempered, and emotionally distant. She stated that although her husband was "a good patient" and was monitoring his diet and sugar, "he acted like a stranger." After several sessions, the husband began to open up about his fears of death, future complications that could occur, and sexual difficulties. Once he shared these feelings, she felt immediately closer to him. ("I feel like I have my husband back.") Subsequent sessions were spent creating a new level of commitment between the couple, one in which the husband was encouraged to show his vulnerability and fears.

What is important in this case was that now instead of dealing with the stress of an illness and marital conflicts, the husband was able to focus on both the physical and emotional effect his diabetes was having on him.

Of all the advice many of us are given as children, the lesson that expressing our feelings is a sign of weakness could not be further from the truth. It is widely accepted in the mental health community that many of the emotional conflicts people suffer are a result of holding in feelings. Depression, anxiety, panic attacks, and sleep disorders are just some of the conflicts that can result from holding in feelings.

Although men tend to express feelings less than women, women can often be less expressive than they need to be. Many men were told as children that crying is a weakness, it shows vulnerability, and it is unattractive to women.

One major reason *psychotherapy* is effective is that it allows people to identify and express their feelings in a safe environment. Psychotherapy also encourages people to take these new skills with them into their day-to-day lives. When people open up to spouses, children, and friends, they gain a sense of emotional intimacy (which we will cover later in this chapter).

We all have found ourselves watching news reports in which acts of rage have affected innocent people. Road rage, anger and jealousy among spouses, and school fights are all instances where individuals allow feelings to build up and then displace them on innocent victims. Although these examples are extreme, they illustrate how repressed feelings play out in the real world. It would be naïve to think that when we hold in day to day feelings, they "just go away." The old story of the man who yells at his wife because he had a bad day at work is all too true. Rather than coming home, talking about his day, which would lead to emotional intimacy, the underlying anger actually leads to tension, hurt, and emotional distance.

Rule Number 2: Don't Judge Your Feelings

Case 2: One reason group therapy and support groups are extremely beneficial is that they allow people to hear others who feel the same way. Recently, Joan and I were conducting a group therapy session made up of eight men, ages forty-one to sixty-three, and one of the men was saying how he had cancer fifteen years ago. He spoke in particular about how cancer had almost cost not only his life but his marriage also, as he was angry, closed off emotionally, and displaced these feelings on his wife. Looking back, he could see how he added an unnecessary burden to his illness. Had he allowed his wife to know what he was feeling, they would have gotten closer through the treatment rather than more distant. By sharing his experience with the group, other men opened up about how they too have "sucked it up" during difficult times rather than "opened it up."

If we look at case 1, one reason the husband held back from sharing with his wife was that he felt he should be able to "handle" it on his own. This is a belief I hear a lot, mostly among men, a belief that puts a tremendous burden on them. Women are much more comfortable sharing their fears and vulnerabilities. My experience as a therapist for the past thirty years is that women handle illness and the emotions that go along with it in a far healthier manner. Women, for the most part, not only want to talk about their feelings, but typically they talk to friends as well as family, thus meeting their emotional needs on a regular basis. It is rare to encounter a man who doesn't judge his vulnerable side as "weak" or "unmanly." This judgment discourages men from opening up to their spouses, and few men will share vulnerable feelings with friends for fear of being judged.

When men share feelings, they tend to be feelings of joy, such as hugging after their team scores a touchdown, or anger, such as acting out when they are cut off by another driver on the road. It is my belief that if men would be more expressive on a day to day basis, heart attacks, strokes, ulcers, and other medical conditions would decline among men. *It cannot be stressed enough that during times of physical illness, the last thing people need to do is judge how they are feeling emotionally.* It is imperative that patients be verbal, open, and allow themselves to express their healthy fears and anxieties.

Rule Number 3: Create Intimacy

Case 3: I was seeing a forty-seven-year-old woman in both individual and group therapy. She initially came in for marriage issues, as she did not feel close to her husband. This particular woman was the exception to the rule: she did not open up emotionally; she was emotionally "hard," and other members of the group described her as acting more like a man than a woman. She was resistant to talking about her feelings and resisted when it came to relating to others.

Coincidentally, she received a phone call from her doctor telling her about her breast cancer literally minutes before our group session started. The timing couldn't have been better, as she started the group by telling everyone what she was told, then immediately broke down and cried, saying how scared she was. She was fearful that she might die, and she questioned how she would share this news with her husband and son. The group was very supportive; they related how it was okay to be scared and allowed her to express herself in whatever way she needed. The following week, in group, she said that had she been told about her cancer at any other time, she would have kept her feelings to herself, cried alone, and not even let her husband know the full extent of her fears. Fortunately, as she went through her treatment, she opened up emotionally, which made it all much more bearable for her. Happily, her cancer was caught early, and she is doing well.

The word "relate" is part of the word relationship, and without the openness and willingness to share emotionally, intimacy does not occur. The ability to create emotional intimacy is essential in order to feel love, closeness, caring, and support.

People going through illness often feel isolated from others, alone in their struggle to deal with the difficult choices that lie ahead. It is common for people to want to isolate themselves, to hide behind a wall of anger, denial, and hurt. This is particularly true during stressful times, and if men do share feelings, they are typically feelings of anger.

The first step to intimacy is trust. People hold in feelings due to past experiences of being hurt. These past experiences usually go back to childhood. Whether by family or friends, they felt abandoned in their time of need. It should be stressed that good listening skills on the part of the spouse or significant other are essential in allowing feelings to be expressed openly. Being a non-judgmental listener will encourage the continued flow of communication and sharing.

Emotional intimacy can occur only when people can let go of these past experiences and begin to trust those close to them. Let's look at an example. A person comes home from a doctor's visit and shares "all about it" with their spouse. They talk about how long they had to wait before seeing the doctor, the examination, any tests that were performed, etc. One might assume that this couple has a great level of communication and knows everything about what occurred at the doctor's visit. Although it is true that all the "facts" were talked about, not one *feeling* was shared. In order to achieve emotional intimacy, the following statements would help:

- "I was really nervous about the appointment."
- "It scares me when I think about getting the tests results back."
- "I feel out of control."
- "Why is this happening to me?"

It is important that we do not take ourselves out of what I call "the human experience," the natural, normal feelings we all experience as human beings. To deny our feelings is to negate a major aspect as who we are as people.

The impact of holding in feelings on our physical illness cannot be measured by a CAT scan or an MRI. However, through self-reports, it is clear that those people who share feelings on a regular basis feel better.

Rule 4: Know Your Personality

Case 4: A fifty-two-year-old woman entered therapy stating she had completed her course of treatment for breast cancer; however, she could not stop obsessing over the possibility of getting cancer again. She was also second guessing her decision not to take tamoxifen. As I got to know her, I soon realized that this was a woman who strived for perfection in everything she did. She was often hard on herself if her cooking wasn't great, put herself down if she made any mistakes, wouldn't go to the grocery store without makeup, and had to keep her house spotless. She stated her husband had pointed out to her "all the time" how much tension he often felt while being around her, as she would "make suggestions" about everything he did. Through therapy, she was able to become less "anal," and as we focused on other areas of her life, her obsession with her cancer subsided significantly.

There are many different personality types listed in the Diagnostic and Statistical Manual of Mental Disorders,[317] the major reference guide in the mental health field. For simplicity's sake, we are going to look at general personality patterns and the effects they have on us.

By "know your personality," I mean that we need to know how we react and feel in various situations. It is important to stress that an examination of "who we are" does not include how we *want* to be seen (our image), or how we act in front of others, but rather our "real self." Are we controlling, dependent, insecure, perfectionist, obsessive compulsive, etc.? How does who we really are affect us and the people around us? How many people "really know us"? How much effort do we put into hiding our real selves? Do people see more about us than we think they do? One of the many benefits of group therapy is that we get to hear honest feedback about how people experience us—often

---

317   allpsych.com/disorders/dsm.html.

times it is very different from what we think. By being honest with ourselves about who we really are, we can learn the effect our personality has on coping with illness, stress, and interpersonal relationships. One way for people to "know themselves" is to ask for feedback from those close to them, and to take that feedback in an open, non-defensive manner. Obviously, psychotherapy is another way for people to better understand themselves. For example, someone who has the need to be in control will have a more difficult time dealing with all the "out of control" feelings they might experience during an illness or emotional conflict. An obsessive compulsive personality may find herself unable to concentrate on anything other than her illness, or may constantly find herself researching every treatment available. The perfectionist may find himself unable to choose a treatment, or a doctor, as his need to make the "perfect" decision paralyzes his.

Rule 5: Avoid Denial

Case 5: A forty-seven-year-old man entered therapy due to generalized anxiety. He stated that several times a day, "for no reason," his heart would race, his palms would get sweaty, and he would feel dizzy. He had been examined by his physician, who cleared him medically and suggested he seek therapy. As his time in therapy progressed, it became apparent that this was a man who rarely knew what a feeling was. He was an only child, doted on by his mother, had "an easy life," and rarely had to deal with emotional conflicts. Three years ago, he left the family business and was now working for an employer. He often found his boss difficult to deal with but never confronted him when he disagreed. He was denied a raise he was promised when he was hired, yet he said nothing. A coworker was given an assignment that he was supposed to get, yet he still remained silent.

We constructed a timeline of events and compared it to his first and subsequent panic attacks, and it became apparent that his passivity at work was playing out emotionally. Through therapy, he began expressing himself to his boss, became more assertive, and noticed his anxiety lessened significantly. He also realized that because he was protected by his parents, he never had to deal with many real-life conflicts. He now felt he had the tools to express himself, and he rarely experienced panic attacks or significant anxiety.

Freud stated that psychological conflicts were often circuitous, meaning that issues could show up as one conflict but could be caused by something totally unrelated. An example would be someone experiencing a panic attack when stuck in traffic. Although they may try to avoid these situations, the real cause of the panic attacks is likely repressed feelings of anger, loss of control, or childhood conflicts. Once again, when we are unaware of or unwilling to explore our inner feelings, these feelings do not just go away; they often surface in other areas of our lives. It is extremely important for us to learn to identify and express feelings on a daily basis.

In the field of psychology, we focus on three important aspects: our thoughts, our feelings, and our behaviors. We know that how we think affects how we feel. We also know that how we feel affects how we think and the decisions that we make. I'll use this example: You are driving, and someone cuts in front of you. You get angry, honk your horn, and yell. As you get closer to the other car, you realize that it is someone you know. Immediately the anger goes away, because your feelings have changed due to your thinking.

Another common example of our thoughts affecting our behavior and feelings is hypochondriasis. People who obsess over their health often create aches and pains that have no physical basis. Someone who experiences a strong headache may think, "I must have a brain tumor" and may actually experience more and more headaches. These people will then become anxious, visit doctors, have tests performed, and often not accept that there is nothing wrong with them physically. Others will find a sense of comfort knowing that no tumor exists, and will move on with their lives.

In order for people to avoid denial, it is once again helpful to ask those close to us for their experience of how they perceive our behaviors, moods, and reactions. All too often people have a perception of themselves that may differ from how others see them.

Rule 6: Seek Help

Case 6: A fifty-five-year-old woman came to see me, stating that she wanted help getting her husband into therapy. He recently had open heart surgery, was no longer working, and seemed to be depressed. He told her that there was no way that he would "talk to a stranger" and that if she wanted to, she should go alone. She told him she would, as she felt she needed help dealing with him. He then complained to her about how much therapy would cost, but she did it anyway. I complimented her on her resolve and set out to help her accomplish her goal of getting her husband into therapy. It was not easy, but through her persistence, he finally showed up "to help her." Surprisingly, after about fifteen minutes, he opened up to both of us about how he felt his "life was over," that he was too old to start any hobbies, and that he felt worthless since his surgery. He agreed to make another appointment, this time without his wife, and began weekly sessions. He eventually started to play golf, took some adult education classes, and over time began to feel better emotionally.

Although psychotherapy is more accepted today than ever before, a judgment still exists. Some people feel they should be able to "fix" their own problems. Seeking help is seen as "weak" and paying someone to listen is like "buying a friend." It is difficult for many to overcome these judgments, but it is important that people experiencing emotional conflicts or serious illness receive the help and support they need. This is where the role of family, friends, and physicians become essential. We must encourage those who need psychotherapy the opportunity to push past their judgments and see a therapist. It has been my experience that once someone actually goes to therapy, they realize it isn't such a "bad thing."

Summary

We need time to think, feel, and understand the effects our world has on us. Only by communicating with one another on an emotional level will we be as happy and healthy as possible. We cannot always change the events around us, but we can certainly maintain emotional closeness with those who are important to us. The key to both physical and emotional health is to keep our feelings at the surface, and our level of communication open. Identifying feelings, communicating with those close to us, and creating intimacy are all essential steps in coping with illness and maintaining mental health. As is evident in these case studies, people cope better, feel less stressed, and are happier when issues are addressed and talked about openly. We can't always control our physical health; however, we can control how we deal with our emotions.

Chapter 15

The Importance of a Health Advocate

People commonly hire personal trainers to assist in physical workouts, life coaches to reach business and personal goals, and dietitians to help with weight loss. The concept of obtaining a healthcare advocate seems far overdue. When patients face overwhelming decisions having to do with treatment choices, it may seem obvious that having an expert to guide them through the process would reduce anxiety and add much needed knowledge to the decision making process. Often, physicians suggest more than one treatment, and they often disagree. A healthcare advocate can advise a patient of the research that exists on treatment protocols, and also act as a liaison between patient and physician to ensure clear communication and understanding of all options. All too often physicians speak in terms that the average patient may not fully understand, complicating the decision making process and adding unnecessary anxiety. There are a number of healthcare advocate associations that you can find online. In addition, we, the authors of this book, are healthcare advocates and may be reached at kreisbergandassociates. com.

Another benefit of a healthcare advocate is objectivity. As much as family and friends try to assist, it is difficult for those close to us to be objective and to remove the emotions that come along when a loved one faces major healthcare choices. A healthcare advocate objectively examines all options available, reviews the most current research available, and makes suggestions based on empirical data. Although at times the choices may not be clear cut, the input received often reduces anxiety, as knowledge adds to a sense of control.

With hundreds of billions of dollars spent on healthcare, it seems logical to accept that spending money "out of pocket" for a healthcare advocate could actually save money in the long run. Unnecessary tests and doctor visits could be avoided, and only the most proven treatments would be chosen, resulting in safe, quality healthcare. Healthcare advocates offer one more advantage that the patient has in their fight to get well and stay well.

Appendix

Important Phone Numbers and Web Sites

CHAPTER 1: TAKE CONTROL OF YOUR DOCTOR'S APPOINTMENT

- Finding the right doctor: go to the American Board of Medical Specialties, absm.org, healthgrades.com, or ucomparehealth.com

CHAPTER 2: TAKE CONTROL OF YOUR STAY IN THE HOSPITAL

- Joint Commission certifies hospital programs such as addiction/substance abuse, cancer care, diagnostic tests/services, developmental disabilities (hospital, program/services), end-of-life care (including palliative), genetics, health and wellness, women's health, mental health care, hospice, shelter, nursing home care, occupational therapy, spinal care, prosthetics, pediatrics wheelchairs, crutches, and mobility equipment. For certification of your hospital, go to **qualitycheck.org** or **medicare.gov. For comparisons of hospitals in your area, go to** Healthgrades.gov.

The following sites allow you to compare your hospital with others in your area as well as with nationwide averages on key treatments:
- o qualitycheck.org,
- o hospitalcompare.hhs.gov/Hospital/Search/Welcome. asp?version=default&browser=IE percent7C7 percent7C WinXP&language=English&defaultstatus=0&pagelist=Home.
- Hospital death rates from heart attack, heart failure, and pneumonia can be compared by visiting, hospitalcompare.hhs.gov/hospital/mortalitytool/index.asp.

- For a list of hospitals that have volunteered to put their quality data online go, to qualitynet.org. If your hospital has not allowed this information to become public, you may want to consider going to another hospital.
- For a list of recommended treatments go to, hospitalcompare.hhs. gov/Hospital/Static/ConsumerInformation_tabset.asp?activeTab=2 &Language=English&version=default&subTab=4
- For patient safety requirements visit, the National Quality Forum at nqf.org or ahrq.gov.
- To see how your hospital compares to others in preventing falls, go to qualitycheck.org.
- To see the Joint Commission's Standards to reduce hospital error, visit apsf.org/resource_center/newsletter/2001/fall/08jcaho.htm.
- The Patient Safety and Quality Improvement Act of 2005 (Patient Safety Act) is intended to spur the development of voluntary, provider-driven initiatives to improve the quality, safety, and outcomes of patient care, visit, ahrq.hhs.gov/qual/nhqr07/Chap1.htm.
- Medicare's Never Event List, cms.hhs.gov/apps/media/press/release. asp?Counter=1863.
- Types of communication problems that result in medical errors, psqh.com/enews/0708b.shtml
- For tips to stay safe in the hospital visit, cancerlynx.com.

CHAPTER 3: TAKE CONTROL OF YOUR MEDICATIONS
- Pill Card template, go to ahrq.gov/qual/pillcard/pillcard. htm#Template.

Name	Used for	Instructions	Morning	Afternoon	Evening	Night

- For side effects and drug interactions go to fda.gov.
- For over-the-counter drugs to avoid during pregnancy, go to consumerreports.org/health/prescription-drugs/10-over-the-counter-drugs-to-avoid-during-pregnancy/overview/10-over-the-counter-drugs-to-avoid-during-pregnancy-ov.htm.
- For a list of dangerous medications that have been prescribed "off-label" (for conditions for which they're not approved) go to drugtopics. modernmedicine.com/drugtopics/Modern+Medicine+Now/Off-label-drugs-prescribed-without-clinical-eviden/ArticleStandard/Article/detail/578172?contextCategoryId=47448.
- For a list of drugs that can interact with alcohol go to alcoholism. about.com/cs/alerts/l/blnaa27.htm.
- For a list of drugs that can interact with food go to fda.gov/cder/consumerinfo/druginteractions.htm.
- For a list of drug and disease interactions, go to merck.com/mmhe/sec02/ch013/ch013c.html.
- For a list of drug-dietary supplement interactions go to merck.com/mmhe/sec02/ch019/ch019a.html#tb019_1.
- For a list of drug to drug interactions go to merck.com/mmhe/sec02/ch013/ch013c.html.

CHAPTER 4: TAKE CONTROL OF YOUR HEALTH INSURANCE
- To choose a plan that's right for you and your family go to:
  - o naic.org/state.web.htm to find the Web site of your state's insurance regulator.

- o ncqa.org,
- o jointcommission.org,
- o planforyourhealth.com/about/insurance101 or
- o dol.gov/ebsa/publications/10working4you.html
- For a list and rating of private insurance plans go to:
  - o ehealthinsurance.com, ncqa.org
  - o health.usnews.com/sections/health/health-plans/index. html
- For the best health insurance plans go to http://health.usnews.com/ sections/health/health-plans/index.html
- For information on the federal employee health insurance program go to fepblue.gov.
- For Tricare go to military.com/benefits/tricare.
- For Medicare, Medicaid, COBRA, and CHIP, visit cms.gov or call 1-800-MEDICARE.
- For your state's requirements, go to benefits.gov or call 1-800-543-7669.
- For the state's requirements for Medicaid/ SCHIP go to benefits. gov.
- For frequently asked questions about Medicare, Medicaid, COBRA, and SCHIP go to coverageforall.org/ or 1-800-234-1317.
- SCHIP, frequently asked questions: ncsl.org/print/health/forum/ SCHIPFAQ.pdf.
- For questions about the Economic Recovery and Investment Act 2009 go to recovery.gov.
- For information about Community Health Centers go to nachc. com.
- If you've recently lost your job and are searching for insurance go to coverageforall.org/ or call 1-800-234-1317.
- To determine the quality of your health insurance plan go to:
  - o The National Committee for Quality Assurance (NCQA), ncqa.org,
  - o The Joint Commission on Accreditation of Healthcare Organizations (JCAHO) at jointcommission.org.
- To appeal an HMO's decision, go to bankrate.com/brm/news/ insurance/20050726a1.asp.
- To find examples of appeal letters, go to appeallettersonline.com/.
- To find your state's regulatory agency that oversees insurance, go to kff.org.
- To find a health advocacy organization to help with medical claims go to carecounsel.net.

CHAPTER 5: TAKE CONTROL OF YOUR HEALTHCARE: FOR SENIORS

Section 1: Find the Right Doctor and Get the Right Care

- To find a primary care doctor or gerontologist in your area visit absm. org or healthgrades.com.
- To find physicians and other healthcare professionals who participate in Medicare go to:
    - medicare.gov/Physician/Home.asp
    - advocatehealth.com/system/info/library/sam/031204.html

Section 2: Take Control of Your Prescription Medications

- To create a Pill Card to list your medications, go to ahrq.gov/qual/ pillcard/pillcard.htm#Template.
- For a Medicare prescription drug plan finder visit medicare.gov.
- There are forty-one drugs that are potentially dangerous to senior adults and should be avoided. For a list of these drugs go to dcri. duke.edu/curtis/beers.html.
- For a list of potentially dangerous drug-to-drug and drug-dietary supplement interactions, go to
    - merck.com/mmhe/sec02/ch019/ch019a.html#tb019_1
    - merck.com/mmhe/sec02/ch013/ch013c.html
    - aging-parents-and-elder-care.com/Pages/Prescription_ Drugs.html
- For a list of adverse drug-to-alcohol interactions go to alcoholism. about.com/cs/alerts/l/blnaa27.htm.

Section 3: Understand Medicare and Medicaid

- Understanding Medicare and Medicaid, go to:
    - cms.gov
    - carepathways.com/MedicareCoverage.cfm
- For a copy of "Medicare and You 2009," call 1-800-MEDICARE.
- To keep up to date about changes in Medicare visit medicarenewswatch. com.
- For assistance paying for prescription drug coverage or prescription drug, call 1-800-MEDICARE, or go to the National Conference of

State Legislatures (ncsl.org/programs/health/SPAPCCoordination. htp).

- For top Medicare Advantage and Medicaid Plans, visit usnews. com/directories/health-plans/index_html/plan_cat+commercial/ or todaysmedicare.com/.
- Know your rights: visit medicare.gov.
  - o Please visit this site for more information about fast-track reviews, including the service termination notices that providers will deliver, and answers to frequently asked questions. See cms.hhs.gov/MMCAG.
- Medicare Prescription Drug Appeals & Grievances page on cms.gov Web site: cms.hhs.gov/MedPrescriptDrugApplGriev.

Section 4: Take Control of Your Long Term Care

- Long-term care resources:
  - o Go to www.medicare.gov and select, "Plan for your long-term care needs."
  - o Skilled nursing: helpguide.org/elder/nursing_homes_ skilled_nursing_facilities.htm.
  - o Call 1-800-MEDICARE. TYY should call 1-877-486-2048.
  - o Get a copy of the "Own your future planning kit" by visiting longtermcare.gov.
  - o Visit Eldercare Locator at eldercare.gov (or call 1-800-677-1116) to find the Aging and Disability Resource Center in your area. Eldercare is a free public service from the U.S. Administration on Aging.
  - o Resources by state: seniorresource.com/house.htm.
  - o leapfroggroup.org.
- To see if you qualify for Medicaid for long-term care, call 1-800-MEDICARE.
- Call your state insurance department to get more information about long-term care insurance. For that phone number, call, 1-800-MEDICARE.
- Long-term care insurance: For information about policies that meet your need, call the National Association of Insurance Commissioners at 1-866-470-6242 for a copy of "A Shopper's Guide to Long-term Care Insurance," or go to seniorresource.com/insur.htm#long.
- Elder care locator
  - o Eldercarelocator.gov, or call 1-800-677-1116. Eldercare is a

free public service from the U.S. Administration on Aging.
  o nia.nih.gov: "There's No Place Like Home—For Growing Old"
- What you need to know about Advanced Directives
  o neca.org
  o familydoctor.org/online/famdocen/home/pat-advocacy/endoflife/003.printerview.html
- Staying safe: Information on how to protect yourself from falls:
  o healthystates.csg.org/Publications
  o cdc.gov/ncipc/duip/preventadultfalls.htm
  o The Department of Education provides a Web site, abledata.com, with information on more than 30,000 technology products designed to make life easier and safer for people with physical limitations. No computer? Call 1-800-227-0216.
- For home- and community-based services:
  o eldercare.gov/Eldercare.NET/Public/Home.aspx
  o Geriatric Care Manager, caremanager.org
  o familycaregivingonline.org
  o National Association on Area Agencies on Aging, n4a.org/programs/eldercare-locator/ or call 1-202-872-0888
  o Be sure the services you require meets Medicare's quality measures. To find out how agencies rate in your area go to medicare.gov/HHCompare/Home.asp?dest=NAV|Home|About#TabTop or go to eldercarelink.com/
- For independent and assisted living facilities and nursing homes and Alzheimer's units:
  o helpguide.org/elder/adult_day_care_centers.htm
  o Assisted living federation of America, alfa.org
  o American Association of Homes and Services for the Aging (AASHA), aahsa.org/consumer_info
  o cms.gov
- For the worst nursing homes, cms.hhs.gov/CertificationCompliance/downloads/SFFList.pdf
- Resolving disputes that arise in long-term care facilities, seek an ombudsman. Go to the National Long-Term Care Ombudsman Resource Center's Web site: ltcombudsman.org/static_pages/ombudsmen.cfm.
- Palliative and Hospice Care
  o nhpco.org/files/public/Statistics_Research/NHPCO_facts-

and-figures_2008.pdf
- o alz.org/carefinder/careoptions/options1.asp
- o suttervnaandhospice.org/services/services_hospicemyths.
html
- National Hospice Foundation guide: caringinfo.org/userfiles/file/
pdfs/hospiceCare/hospice_care(1).pdf.
- Care for the care giver:
  - o For a few hours of relief, find senior day care. Call the Area
Agency on Aging (1-800-677-1116 for the AAA in your
area), or visit helpguide.org/elder/adult_day_care_centers.
htm.

CHAPTER 7: TAKE CONTROL OF HEART DISEASE
- Risk factors for heart disease
  - o Risk factor calculator, hin.nhlbi.nih.gov/atpiii/calculator.
asp?usertype=prof
  - o BMI calculator: nytimes.com/ref/health/bmi.html
- USPSTF screening recommendations
  - o ahrq.gov/clinic/uspstf/uspsacad.htm (coronary artery
disease)
  - o ahrq.gov/clinic/uspstf/uspshype.htm (high blood pressure)
- Best practice guidelines for heart attack
  - o mayoclinic.com/health/coronary-artery-disease/DS00064/
DSECTION=treatments-and-drugs
  - o hrq.gov/research/tripcad.htm
- Heart attack symptoms in men and women
  - o mayoclinic.com/health/heart-attack/DS00094/
DSECTION=symptoms
- For designated best heart hospitals, go to
  - o jointcommission.org/CertificationPrograms/Disease-
SpecificCare/DSCOrgs
- For the warning signs of cardiac arrest, go to
  - o mayoclinic.com/health/sudden-cardiac-arrest/DS00764
- Dietary fat recommendations, go to
  - o americanheart.org/presenter.jhtml?identifier=532
  - o Fish oil: americanheart.org/presenter.jhtml?identifier=4632
  - o http://www.ahrq.gov/clinic/uspstfab.htm
- For help in finding a cardiologist, go to absm.org, healthgrades.com,
or ucomparehealth.com

CHAPTER 8: TAKE CONTROL OF HYPERTENSION

o Guidelines for hypertension:
o The "Seventh Report of the Joint National Committee on Prevention, Detection, Evaluation, and Treatment of High Blood Pressure" nhlbi.nih.gov/guidelines/hypertension/ or mayoclinic.com/health/high-blood-pressure/HI99999

CHAPTER 9: TAKE CONTROL OF STROKE

- What you should know about stroke-risk factors, symptoms, prevention, and treatments
  o stroke.org/site/PageNavigator/HOME
  o mayoclinic.com/health/stroke/DS00150
  o strokeassociation.org/presenter.jhtml?identifier=1020
  o mayoclinic.com/health/stroke/DS00150/DSECTION=symptom
  o americanstrokeassociation.org/presenter.jhtml?identifier=1200037
- Find a hospital in your area that is a designated stroke center. *This is a matter of life and death*:
  o You can find a stroke center in your area by visiting jointcommission.org/CertificationPrograms/Disease-SpecificCare/DSCOrgs, and look under "Primary stroke centers."
  o Or visit stroke.org/site/DocServer/Stroke_Center_List.pdf?docID=1741. In most areas, there are no uniform guidelines for 9-1-1 dispatch and emergency medical service to get patients to a hospital that can provide the treatment they need. *Demand that your ambulance driver take you to a stroke center.*
- For information about stroke from rehabilitation to nursing homes and assisted living, to insurance questions and financial assistance, to support groups and other questions, visit the National Stroke Association and Resource Directory at stroke.org/site/PageServer?pagename=Resource_Directory_list
  o You can also call 1-888-4-STROKE (478-7653) and ask for the Stroke Family Support Network.
- Tips for Caregivers: Please see "Caregiver Journal Pages" at strokeassociation.org/presenter.jhtml?identifier=3042556.

CHAPTER 10: TAKE CONTROL OF DIABETES

- For information about risk factors, symptoms, prevention, associated risks, and treatment see:

- mayoclinic.com/health/diabetes/DS01121
- diabetes.org
- stroke.org/site/PageNavigator/HOME
- For a symptom check-up, go to mayoclinic.com/health/symptom-checker/DS00671.
- To calculate your risk for developing diabetes, go to diabetes.org/risk-test.jsp
- Screening and diagnosis of diabetes:
  - professional.diabetes.org/Disease_Backgrounder. aspx?MID=233&RD=1
  - ahrq.gov/clinic/uspstf/uspsdiab.htm
  - diabetes.niddk.nih.gov/dm/pubs/diagnosis/#3
- To determine your BMI, go to bmi-calculator.net.
- For a calorie counter, go to nytimes.com/ref/health/caloriecounter. html.
- For information on managing the disease, go to mayoclinic.com.
- For primary prevention interventions, seek to delay or halt the development of diabetes.
- For secondary and tertiary prevention interventions, focus on people with diabetes and seek to prevent (secondary) or control (tertiary) the devastating complications of this disease, go to healthierus.gov/steps/summit/prevportfolio/strategies/reducing/diabetes/prevention.htm.
- Metabolic syndrome: mayoclinic.com/health/metabolic percent20syndrome/DS00522.

CHAPTER 11: TAKE CONTROL OF CANCER

- For definitions of the different terms used in cancer, go to cancer.net/patient/Learning+About+Cancer
- For a cancer specialist go to abms.org
- **For a Cancer Center**, visit nci.nih.gov
- **Treatment options** for 70 percent to 80 percent of cancers can be found at the National Cancer Comprehensive Network at nccn.org
- Cervical cancer
  - cancer.net/patient/Cancer+Types/Cervical+Cancer
  - preventiveservices.ahrq.gov
  - HPV vaccine, guidelines.gov/summary/summary. aspx?doc_id=11876
- Breast cancer
  - cancer.net/patient/Cancer+Types/Breast+Cancer
  - qap.sdsu.edu/screening/breastcancer/facts.html
  - preventiveservices.ahrq.gov

- o information on sentinel biopsy
- o cancer.net/patient/ASCO+Resources/What+to+Know percent3A+ASCO percent27s+Guidelines/What+to+Know percent3A+ASCO percent27s+Guideline+on+Sentinel+Lymph+Node+Biopsy+in+Early+Stage+Breast+Cancer
- o National Cancer Institute Breast Cancer Risk Tool (the "Gail model") go to
- o cancer.gov/bcrisktool or call 1-800-4-CANCER.
- Skin cancer
  - o Non-melanoma cancer.net/patient/Cancer+Types/ Skin+Cancer+ percent28Non-Melanoma percent29
  - o Melanoma
  - o cancer.net/patient/Cancer+Types/Melanoma
- Colorectal cancer (cancer of the colon and rectum)
  - o cancer.net/patient/Cancer+Types/Colorectal+Cancer
  - o screening/prevention
  - o ahrq.gov/clinic/uspstf/uspscolo.htm
  - o American College of Gastroenterology Guidelines for Colorectal Cancer Screening 2008 Am J Gastroenterol 104: 739, 2009
- Prostate cancer
  - o cancer.net/patient/Cancer+Types/Prostate+Cancer
  - o There is a clinical trial taking place that will determine the benefits of PSA and DRE screening, but the results will not be known for several years.
  - o cancer.gov/cancertopics/factsheet/PLCOProstateFactSheet
- Endometrial cancer
  - o The American Cancer Society recommends that all menopausal women should be informed about the risks and symptoms of endometrial cancer, and strongly encouraged to report any unexpected bleeding or spotting to their doctors. For women with or at high risk for hereditary non-polyposis colon cancer (HNPCC), annual screening should be offered for endometrial cancer with endometrial biopsy beginning at age thirty-five.
  - o cancer.org/docroot/CRI/content/CRI_2_4_3X_Can_ endometrial_cancer_be_found_early.asp?sitearea=
  - o General information about clinical trials is available from the National Cancer Institute Web site, cancer.gov/ clinicaltrials.
  - o To interpret prognostic factors go to, adjuvantonline.com.

The information presented here should be used with your doctor's guidance.

Chapter 12: Take Control of Chronic Obstructive Pulmonary Disease

- copdguide.com/copd-is-different.asp
- Compare and contrast asthma and COPD: aarc.org/klein/what_is_copd.asp

Chapter 13: Take Control of Dementia

- Facts about Alzheimer's Disease:
  - alzheimer.ca/english/disease/faqs.htm
  - health.nytimes.com/ref/health/healthguide/esn-alzheimers-ess.
  - alz.org/alzheimers_disease_facts_figures.asp
- Specialists: For the names of a geriatrician, or geriatric psychiatrist, see abms.com.
- For a geriatric care manager, go to caremanager.org.
- Risk factors for developing Alzheimer's disease, visit:
  - Alz.org
  - Health.nytimes.com/health/guides/disease/alzheimers-disease/overview.html?print=1
  - newswise.com/articles/view/539441/?sc=dwhr
  - cnn.com/2009/HEALTH/01/26/health.calories.memory
- Symptoms of Alzheimer's disease: Alz.org
- What to ask your doctor about Alzheimer's disease:
  - New York Times, health.nytimes.com/ref/health/healthguide/esn-alzheimers-ask.html
  - Alzheimer's Association, alz.org
  - Alzheimer's Society, www.alzheimer.ca/english/disease/faqs.htm
- Exams and tests
  - Alzheimer's Association, alz.org
  - National Institute on Aging, nia.nih.gov
- Prognosis
  - Alzheimer's Association, alz.org
  - National Institute of Neurological Disorders and Stroke , ninds.nih.gov
- Treatment of Alzheimer's

- o Non-drug approaches
- Alzheimer's Association, alz.org
- Alzheimer's Society, www.alzheimer.ca/english/disease/faqs.htm
  - o Drug approaches
- Alzheimer's Association, alz.org/alzheimers_disease_standard_ prescriptions.asp
- Alzheimer's Society, www.alzheimer.ca/english/disease/faqs.htm
- *Wall Street Journal*, wsj.com/article/SB123603689949914421.html
- Setting up home care
  - o helpguide.org/elder/alzheimers_disease_dementias_caring_ caregivers.htm
  - o Alzheimer's Association, alz.org/national/documents/book_ coachbroylesplaybook.pdf
  - o For advice, support, information, or referrals, call 1-866-232-8484
  - o "Guidelines for Care" (for a free copy of the booklet, contact your local Alzheimer's Society)
- Finding adult day care services
  - o National Institute on Aging, Niapublications.org/pubs/ long-distance/So_Far)Away_Twenty_Questions_For_ Long_Distance_Caregivers.pdf
  - o helpguide.org
  - o Benefitscheckup.org
  - o Alzheimer's Association, alz.org
  - o Alzheimer's Society, www.alzheimer.ca/english/disease/faqs. htm4
- Finding the best Alzheimer's facilities
  - o Alzheimer's Association, alz.org
  - o Alzheimer's Society, alzheimer.ca/english/disease/faqs.htm
  - o helpguide.org/elder/alzheimers_disease_dementias_caring_ caregivers.htm helpguide.org
  - o Eldercare Locator—national resource to find support groups, care giving in your area: http://www.eldercare.gov/ Eldercare.NET/Public/Network/Network.aspx
  - o Gilbert's Guide, gilbertguide.com
  - o American Association of Homes and Services for the Aging, aahsa.org
  - o Leapfroggroup.org